Green Renaissance

Green Renaissance

Unveiling the Historical Influence of Cannabis on Wellness, Lifestyle, and Culture Worldwide

JM Balbuena

Cover design by Savina Monet
Editor: Andrae Smith, Lantern Literary LLC
Graphics by Proud Mary Network
Author's photo courtesy of Thais Brown
Cover photo by Yanira Amaya

Contents

For my uncle, Tío Julito, I love you and miss you dearly.

Foreword
Terrie Best

"High, Queen!

Thank you so much for your support & most importantly, for all the work & legacy of advocacy in our beloved space!

Love Always, JMB"

These are the words Johann wrote in my copy of her first book, *The Successful Canna-preneur*. In black pen, indelibly, I had earned the respect of this powerhouse and her big, beautiful brain I've come to treasure.

That alone was humbling. But when asked to write a foreword for *Green Renaissance*, Johann's second book, of course I was delighted. Still, that does not describe the humility and honor I felt to be asked.

Johann is an industry professional and a cannabis activist. While that used to be a commonplace and synonymous role, it is no longer so. Legalization in California has changed the landscape, and like any stigmatized, overtaxed, and over-regulated product, competition becomes brutal, and not many celebrate or even advocate for the success of others. Johann does. I wish I could count all the times she has said yes to me when I ask her to show up to help others—mainly elected officials

—learn and thrive in the cannabis and patient advocacy space. Integrity is what comes to mind. Bravery too.

I first met Johann as I was chairing the San Diego Chapter of Americans for Safe Access (ASA), a cannabis patient advocacy group. Most people I agree to meet with want to learn all they can from me with an eye toward entering the market. I seldom meet people with professional knowledge of how to get licensed and permitted. Not because there are none, but because they don't need me, and they know it. Johann didn't need me, and she probably knew that, but that wasn't her aim for the meeting. She learned what I do, and she started supporting our group by attending our monthly meetings and bringing her friends.

One of the more memorable events we arranged was a mayoral forum where we surprised the candidates by asking them to grind some buds and roll joints. We wanted them to understand that every wounded Marine and every grandmother with cancer who wanted natural medicine had to get past their government-induced fear and stigma to simply handle the flower, a natural medicine that cannot harm you. We wanted them to unwrap and use the grinder, get their fingers sticky, and we gave them no assistance. Electeds should know what patients experience.

I see that Johann's intention with this book was to encourage readers to not only get acquainted with this remarkable plant but to solidify its position as a trusted friend to us all. She has woven cannabis history into its quest for freedom in the most comprehensive way, and it is thrilling in its completeness. You will find yourself rooting for our beloved plant. And congratulations! To be a friend of weed, you are rejecting a system being used to perpetuate the school-to-prison pipeline, and you are saying no to "Prohibitionist Profiteers," the enemies of health and justice.

Drug prevention tactics, such as stings and undercovers in high schools, are the drug war. These tactics are still being used and even revered by law enforcement, cheered on by drug preventionists. Sometimes even funded by preventionists. This feeds the school-to-prison pipeline and is heinous. Yet, most lawmakers believe you first must arrest people to prevent their use. And, when it comes to cannabis use —benign at worst, full of wellness and healing at best—it is particularly ugly to criminalize, marginalize and stigmatize cannabis patients.

I hear from Black community members much of their cannabis use was for coping with the realization that their skin color made their lives harder. I can't begin to understand what that feels like, but I can find enough shame and regret for our drug laws to fight fiercely to change them. This book's aim is to make cannabis warriors of us all.

Johann knows that activating others to good causes is a superpower. She seeks to do this in her books, media, and her very essence. She found cannabis to be a great cause, and she will teach you how to be a leader in reducing the stigma. This comes with a deep understanding that cannabis can build power in underserved communities. If politicians could only see that as a revenue stream to channel good. But they funnel too much cannabis-generated income into law enforcement budgets, the one area where no helpful changes happen.

Many times, I have seen our electeds offer the world to over-policed neighborhoods at election time, only to forget them after being elected. There's a saying that goes, "First get elected, then do good." The underlying idea is that they never do the good because their eyes are perpetually in the next election. What if politicians forwarded policies to help equalize and equi-tize income and wealth? Some of that money would go back into helping to elect politicians dedicated to doing more of that. It is an investment, but lawmakers blow it every single time. Let the marginalized into the cannabis economy, and we will do good.

Kicking the door in to let the power lift us all is what the cannabis industry can do for evolution and the advancement of equality. And some cities allow that through cannabis equity programs. I'm in California, and our state cannabis division provides grant money to municipalities that want to launch these programs. Unfortunately, several cities have applied for the first phase, an assessment of who was harmed, but never completed the second, funds to actually make it easier for the identified demographics to engage in the market.

Working to change this has a myriad of benefits. It is a righteous cause, and our plant is up to it. From religious sacrament to medical necessity to earning its "essential" status during the global pandemic—against the backdrop of a brutal political battering—cannabis survived and is thriving. That is because people like Johann are good stewards.

Read the book and refer to it often, for it is a primer and a reference. A must for anyone embarking on a career or advocacy in the times of the cannabis renaissance.

Terrie Best

Co-chair San Diego Chapter of Americans for Safe Access

Chapter 1
Allow me to Re-introduce Myself

High, I'm JM. At the heart of my journey into the fascinating world of cannabis is a simple truth: cannabis is a plant that sprouts from a seed, and it carries properties that are beneficial to both our bodies and the environment. Believe it or not, it's as straightforward as that. So, if this concept rings clear to you, you may not need to peruse the rest of this book. But, if your curiosity spiked up at the thought of how we deviated from such an uncomplicated understanding of cannabis to the convoluted mess we're in today, you're in for a treat. My goal with this book is to provide a comprehensive account built upon meticulous historical research, objective analysis, and personal commentary on the pivotal moments that disrupted the path and muddled things up for anyone possessing an endocannabinoid system.

In case you're unfamiliar with my previous work, I penned a book titled *The Successful Canna-preneur* in 2020. I recommend it to those interested in understanding my beginnings in the cannabis industry and my subsequent evolution in navigating its dynamic landscape. To encapsulate, the cannabis plant played a double role in my life. It was instrumental in my healing process and equally significant in revealing my life's purpose. That purpose is to promulgate the message that's been championed by many before me: that the cannabis plant is inherently good. It carries tremendous potential for our personal well-being, environmental preservation, social justice, and economic prosperity. This rich tapestry of cannabis business, science, culture, and lifestyle stirs something within me, a spark that provokes intrigue and inspires motivation. I find myself immersed in discussions about it, spending countless hours pondering and researching it and consuming it both literally and metaphorically.

My professional journey in cannabis commenced at Prime Harvest Inc., a cannabis organization headquartered in San Diego, CA. My initial role as an assistant to the CEO was multi-faceted, though my understanding of the cannabis industry was quite limited at the onset. My background, coupled with available resources, directed my focus toward the administrative and compliance aspects of the regulated industry. Little did I know, then, this focus on compliance would soon become the cornerstone of my professional identity in the cannabis space. I was instrumental in securing cultivation, manufacturing, and retail licenses for Prime Harvest Inc. and subsequently developing a license acquisition and compliance management department under the guidance of Duane Alexander, the CEO. Our proficiency in the field grew to such an extent that we began consulting with other companies seeking to acquire licenses in CA and several other legal states. From an assistant, I climbed up the ranks to become a shareholder and the current Chief Marketing Officer of Prime Harvest Inc., a journey that, in my opinion, warrants a stand-alone book.

Just like any growing industry, the world of cannabis startups is characterized by intense highs and lows. The ever-changing business environment can exhaust you to the core. I reiterated this in my previous book, and I'll stress it again here: this industry is not for the faint-hearted. My commitment to Prime Harvest Inc. was unwavering, and I worked tirelessly, almost seven days a week, for two straight years during its start-up phase. Recognizing my level of expertise after these grueling years, I made a promise to myself: I would harness this drive and channel it toward crafting my own legacy. This marked the birth of

Balbuena Consulting, a cannabis license acquisition and compliance management organization. In due course, Balbuena Consulting evolved into Synergy as we identified and sought to address other significant challenges in cannabis, including marketing, social equity, and advocacy. Today, Synergy stands as a comprehensive cannabis consultancy and a full-service media production, product integration, and content marketing organization.

Having been in the US cannabis industry for almost a decade, I can attest that running a business in a federally restricted industry is a colossal task. But what's even more challenging is dismantling the massive barrier created by a century of brainwashing, misinformation, criminalization, and discrimination via the War on Drugs and the global criminalization of substance abuse. In my personal mission and my organization's mission, we aim to redefine cannabis advocacy through content marketing, propelling unbiased information about the world of cannabis, and empowering people to make educated decisions about the plant.

A question that's been asked countless times—why is cannabis illegal? The answer to that isn't simple, and that's what this book aims to tackle. Contrary to popular belief, cannabis is a plant that grows flowers and grows from seed. Specifically, the female flowers produce THC, the molecule known for causing its notorious "euphoric" effects. When this same cannabis plant has a low THC content, specifically 0.3% or less in the US, it's referred to as hemp. Hemp, legalized in 2018 in the US, is an incredibly versatile plant that can be used to make a wide array of sustainable commercial and industrial products such as textiles, food, paper, and biofuels.

The distinction between medical and recreational use of cannabis is another issue shrouded in misconceptions. Not too long ago, a long-time customer at Jaxx Cannabis, our dispensary in Southern California, happened to come in just a few weeks after we were awarded the adult-use designation, which would allow us to sell cannabis products to adults over the age of twenty-one. She advised she read somewhere that all dispensaries in our town were now recreational. She expressed concerns about not being considered a medical patient if she shopped with us going forward. I explained that at the core of it, it's the intent of consumption that differentiates the two, not the plant itself. Cannabis, used to alleviate symptoms of a health condition, is deemed for medical use, while the same plant, used because one simply wants to and is of legal age, is considered recreational use. She said she did not think of it that way, but it made complete sense.

This book is not merely about understanding the plant but also about comprehending the wild journey this plant has traversed in our society and how this has influenced our collective psyche and policy-making. My intent is for this book to serve as a tool for cannabis advocates and those willing to learn from our past to shape a more informed future.

The exploration into cannabis history reveals a remarkable narrative filled with a wide array of characters: brave pioneers who dared to use the plant for medical reasons, cunning businessmen who capitalized on its criminalization or its recreational potential, and misguided politicians who sought to control and prohibit it based on misinformation and racial prejudice. Each character has played a part in the plant's convoluted legal status today, and it's our duty to analyze and process their contributions critically and objectively.

Over time, cannabis has endured a constant change of identity. In ancient societies, it was regarded as a sacred herb, revered for its therapeutic properties. Ancient texts from China and India speak volumes about the plant's medicinal use, highlighting its significance in their traditional practices. In the Western world, during the colonial era, hemp was an essential crop that powered economies. It was mandatory in some colonies for farmers to cultivate hemp, such was its significance in the socioeconomic framework of the time.

However, the turn of the twentieth century marked a paradigm shift in the perception of cannabis. It was a time when propaganda against cannabis reached an unprecedented scale. Misinformation was rampant, fueling paranoia and anxiety about the plant's usage. A myriad of factors, including racial prejudice, economic competition, and the need for societal control, coalesced to solidify a negative reputation for the plant. The resultant legal prohibitions only served to exacerbate the situation, culminating in the War on Drugs, a disastrous campaign with significant social consequences to this date.

Today, we stand at a crossroads. On one hand, we have an expanding body of scientific evidence highlighting the benefits of cannabis and a growing legal industry generating billions of dollars in revenue. On the other hand, we continue to witness the detrimental effects of cannabis prohibition, especially on marginalized communities, further deepening the social divide. Navigating this dichotomy calls for a radical shift, a shift that entails a return to our roots, to recognize and acknowledge the inherent influence of this plant in the human experience.

This book seeks to strike a balance between these contrasting perspectives, offering a comprehensive understanding of the cannabis plant in all its glory and infamy. Be prepared to dive into the plant's biology, unraveling the mysteries of cannabinoids and the endocannabinoid system. Plus, examine the vast potential of cannabis as a tool for wellness, understanding how it interacts with our bodies to offer relief from a multitude of ailments.

From there, we then explore the legal landscape of cannabis, examining the patchwork of laws that govern its use across different jurisdictions. This journey takes us across the United States and beyond, showcasing the different models of cannabis legalization and their associated successes and challenges. We also touch upon the burgeoning cannabis industry, shedding light on its economic potential and its implications for social equity. Alongside this, we explore the War on Drugs, examining its historical context, its motivations, and its lasting impact on society.

Last, we look forward to the future of cannabis. A future that promises innovative medical breakthroughs, eco-friendly industrial applications, and a more equitable society. A future where cannabis is not feared but revered for its colorful impact on humanity.

I don't think you will be persuaded by this book to embrace

cannabis. But one thing is for sure, you will feel equip with the knowledge and understanding to conceptualize an informed opinion. Whether you are a patient seeking relief, a parent concerned about your child's exposure to cannabis, a businessperson eyeing the lucrative cannabis market, a policy-maker tasked with regulating its commercial use, or just curious, this book can serve as a reference, offering a balanced perspective on the fascinating topic of cannabis.

Let's get into it!

Chapter 2
Deep Roots: A Prehistoric Perspective

Let's start from the beginning.

All propaganda and stereotypes aside, the cannabis plant has over six thousand years of documented history. The controversial plant, without a doubt, has a compelling global narrative. Its therapeutic applications, it seems, were understood and utilized by a myriad of cultures throughout history. As of March 2024, only Canada, Uruguay, and twenty-four states in the US—including Washington D.C. and Guam—have fully legalized adult-use cannabis. Hence, we find ourselves standing at the cusp of a veritable Green Renaissance, watching as the curtain slowly unfurls, revealing the potentialities of this misunderstood plant.

But this Green Renaissance is not a sudden, unexpected occurrence. It's not a rebellion but a resurgence of ancient wisdom that has been silenced for centuries. Let's make one thing clear: this is no fresh discovery; rather, it is a much-needed reawakening of an old truth that has been buried beneath layers of stigma and misinformation.

Cannabis is not the new kid on the block; it is an old friend slowly but surely returning after a prolonged, unjustified exile, equivalent to the circumstances of those 40,000+ doing time in prison for nonviolent cannabis crimes in the US. Cannabis has deep roots that extend far into the depths of human history, threading through countless cultures and societies, from the tribal communities of prehistoric times to the sophisticated civilizations of the ancient world.

In this chapter, we excavate these roots, venturing on a journey back through time, unraveling the story of cannabis, thread by thread. We unearth evidence of its early uses, exploring its role in religious ceremonies and its recognition as a potent medicinal herb. We voyage across continents, visiting ancient civilizations that valued the plant to understand their relationship with it. Here we go!

8000 BC

The introduction of hemp fiber in Taiwan around 8000 BC represents a significant milestone in the relationship between humanity and the cannabis plant. It is one of the earliest documented instances of humans leveraging the practical benefits of cannabis, particularly hemp, for its utility as a material resource.

As mentioned in the previous chapter, hemp is a variety of the cannabis plant species specifically grown for industrial uses of its derived products. It's one of the fastest-growing plants and was one of the first plants to be spun into usable fiber thousands of years ago.

The discovery of hemp fiber in Taiwan around 8000 BC implies that early civilizations had recognized the plant's utility. The inhabitants of the island might have discovered that the stalk of the cannabis plant, from which hemp fiber is extracted, could be broken down and processed into a durable, versatile material.

The applications of hemp fiber are many and varied. In ancient times, it was often spun into cord or yarn and used to create a variety of objects, including clothing, fishing nets, ropes, and paper. The discovery of hemp fiber use during this period suggests that these early Taiwanese communities were exploring and innovating with available natural resources, contributing to the development of primitive technologies and tools. This demonstrates the integral role that cannabis, in the form of hemp, played in fostering early human industry and craftsmanship.

The early use of hemp fiber in Taiwan also provides valuable insight into the propagation of cannabis across different regions. Its presence in the region around 8000 BC predates its known cultivation in mainland China, indicating the potential for seafaring or migratory dissemination of the plant. This can be interpreted as cannabis in Taiwan during 8000 BC playing a significant role in maritime activities, potentially contributing to early Taiwanese cultures exploring, trade, or fishing more effectively.

This historic introduction of hemp fiber in Asia is not only a testament to the longevity of the human-cannabis relationship but also a reminder of the diverse, practical uses of the plant which extend far beyond the recreational and medicinal applications we often associate with it today. As the modern world reevaluates and navigates its relationship with cannabis, these historical uses of hemp offer a broader perspective on the potential this plant holds.

4000 BC

There is evidence of usage of cannabis around 4000 BC in Pan-p'o Village, currently an archaeological site in China. This is another significant marker in the historical journey of the cannabis plant. During this period, cannabis was classified among the "five grains," which were staples in ancient Chinese agriculture. This classification indicates the central role of cannabis in the economy and culture at the time.

Pan-p'o Village, believed to be one of the oldest agricultural sites in China, thrived in the Neolithic Age, when humans were transitioning from a nomadic existence to settled farming communities. In this context, the cultivation of cannabis was part of an important shift in human society: the transition from a foraging civilization into the organized farming of crops that would sustain the community throughout the year while settled in one location. This shift fundamentally changed the way humans lived, moving from a hunter-gatherer existence to a settled lifestyle that eventually led to the development of civilization as we know it today.

The plant was valued not just for its psychoactive properties, but as a source of food and materials. Hemp seeds, which are highly nutritious, were consumed as food, while the sturdy hemp fibers were used to make a variety of items like clothing, shoes, ropes, and an early form of paper.

The designation of hemp as one of the "five grains" suggests that it was considered a major food crop, alongside staples like rice, millet, barley, and soybeans. This acknowledgment underscores the nutritional importance of cannabis in the ancient Chinese diet and its agricultural value in feeding a growing population.

Moreover, it is a testament to the multifaceted applications of cannabis and hemp—from nourishment to manufacturing materials—all of which made it an integral part of society. This wide usage also suggests a deep understanding of the plant's properties and potential, revealing an early sophistication in agricultural practices.

As we reflect on the historical usage of cannabis, this instance from 4000 BC in Pan-p'o Village helps to contextualize the modern conversation about cannabis. Today, as we explore the medicinal, recreational, and industrial uses of the plant, we're not just innovating; we are also, in many ways, reclaiming a fundamental element of our agricultural past.

2737 BC

The usage of cannabis as medicine can be traced back to 2737 BC under the reign of Emperor Shen Neng in China. Known as one of the earliest fathers of Chinese medicine, Emperor Shen Neng is a legendary figure who significantly shaped ancient Chinese medical theory with his teachings. His guidance about cannabis's medicinal potential signified one of the plant's earliest instances of recorded pharmacology.

Emperor Shen Neng prescribed cannabis as a remedy for a plethora of ailments, revealing his advanced understanding of the plant's therapeutic properties. His application of cannabis as a treatment for conditions such as gout, rheumatism, and malaria was groundbreaking for the time. The concept of using plant-based compounds to treat medical conditions represents the early evolution of medicine in almost every society.

Gout, a form of inflammatory arthritis and rheumatism, referring to a range of conditions affecting the joints and connective tissue, were known to cause intense pain. The emperor's prescription of cannabis for these ailments hints at an early awareness of the plant's pain-relieving properties. This ancient practice echoes in today's use of medical cannabis for chronic pain management.

Similarly, the emperor's recognition of cannabis in treating malaria, a severe and sometimes deadly disease caused by parasites and typically transmitted through mosquito bites, suggests that the emperor recognized the potential of cannabis to alleviate some of the symptoms associated with this condition including fatigue and nausea, symptoms that are known to be manageable with cannabis today.

Ultimately, Emperor Shen Neng's documentation of medicinal use of the plant showcases an ancient understanding of therapeutic practices that have evolved and continue to influence modern medicine today. His knowledge of cannabis and its myriad of uses exemplifies a time-honored connection between human health and the plant-based world. His prescriptions set the stage for thousands of years of medical exploration and use of cannabis and can be directly linked to the twenty-first century's renewed interest in scientific investigation into its medicinal properties.

1550 BC

The Ebers Papyrus, named after George Ebers, the man who purchased it in Luxor, Egypt in 1873, is one of the oldest and most significant medical documents in existence. Dating back to 1550 BC, this comprehensive record reveals a wealth of ancient Egyptian medical knowledge.

Among the wealth of health-related information contained within this ancient document is a notable reference to cannabis as a therapeutic agent. The Ebers Papyrus cites cannabis as a potent treatment for inflammation. This recognition, while primitive by today's standards, demonstrates an ancient understanding of cannabis's anti-inflammatory properties.

Inflammation, the body's response to injury or infection, often results in redness, heat, swelling, and pain. Cannabis, according to the Ebers Papyrus, was recognized as a remedy that could alleviate these symptoms. The inclusion of cannabis in such an ancient medical text highlights not only its therapeutic utility in the past but also underscores the historical continuity of its medical usage.

The Ebers Papyrus is part of a vast archive of ancient records suggesting the utilization of cannabis for various ailments. But it is equally important to note that the mention of cannabis as a remedy for inflammation in this area of the world while in a different century from the one mentioned before, marks a significant recognition of one of the properties we continue to explore in modern medicinal cannabis research. This remarkable testament to early medical wisdom serves as a bridge connecting our current understanding of cannabis to its historical roots.

1400 BC

References to cannabis in the **Atharva Veda** (Sanskrit: अथर्वणवेद:), one of the four sacred texts of Hinduism, illustrated the plant's deep-seated position in society and spirituality. These ancient Hindu religious texts depicted cannabis as a "source of happiness," a "joy-giver," and a "provider of freedom." During this period, the consumption of cannabis wasn't merely an act of individual enjoyment; it was integral to the daily devotional services and religious ceremonies. The cannabis plant was revered and valued not only for its mind-altering effects but also for its deep spiritual significance.

By 1400 BC, the importance of cannabis in Indian culture becomes even more apparent. In the holy book of Atharvana Veda, there are mentions of the plant's anti-anxiety effects, demonstrating another early understanding of its potential therapeutic applications. This period marked open religious use of cannabis, which in turn provided opportunities to explore and understand its medical benefits more extensively. Cannabis was used to treat a wide array of conditions. Among these were ailments such as epilepsy, rabies, and bronchitis. This demonstrates a remarkably sophisticated use of the cannabis plant in medicine in India during ancient times, pointing toward early yet high-level knowledge of its many therapeutic benefits.

The portrayal of cannabis as a sacred plant and its use in medicine during these ancient times set the foundations for the plant's ongoing relationship with humanity. Its use in religious practices, coupled with its recognized therapeutic properties, reflects an early holistic approach to wellness, combining the spiritual, mental, and physical aspects of health. This holistic approach is still relevant today, as modern societies continue to explore and validate the therapeutic potentials of plant and fungi medicine.

1213 BC

The discovery of cannabis pollen on the mummy of Ramesses II, one of Egypt's most powerful and revered pharaohs, who reigned from 1279 BC to 1213 BC, is a significant historical find. It suggests that the Egyptians recognized and utilized the plant's properties centuries ago, perhaps for a variety of uses, from medicinal to ritualistic.

Ramesses II, often regarded as one of Egypt's greatest pharaohs, led several military expeditions, commissioned many architectural feats, and is celebrated for his contributions to the arts. His mummy, discovered in a cache in Deir el-Bahri in 1881 and now displayed in the Cairo Museum, continues to yield insights into the practices and lifestyle of the time.

The presence of cannabis pollen on his mummy indicates that the plant was likely a part of the embalming materials. On one hand, it is plausible to suggest that the Egyptians used cannabis in their mummification processes, likely due to its preservative and insecticidal properties. On the other hand, it is also possible that cannabis was used as part of the burial rituals or, perhaps, as an offering. While the exact reasons remain speculative, the find reaffirms the presence of cannabis in a place where it had to be placed intentionally.

Moreover, this discovery lends credence to the cannabis references found in ancient Egyptian medical texts like the Ebers Papyrus. While the mummy's pollen evidence doesn't provide direct proof of medicinal use, it complements textual references suggesting that cannabis was a part of the Egyptian pharmacopoeia.

The integration of cannabis into such a significant aspect of ancient North African culture (i.e., the death rites of a pharaoh) once again emphasizes its value and versatility in historical contexts. Ramesses II's mummy reminds us that our understanding and use of cannabis is part of a dialogue that spans millennia, cultures, and continents.

600 BC

Located at the crossroads of Europe and Asia, southern Russia has been the cradle of numerous cultures throughout history, each leaving its distinct footprint. Evidence of hemp rope dating back to 600 BC in southern Russia provides compelling evidence of the early widespread use of the plant, specifically the utilitarian applications of its fibers. The use of hemp for making rope places emphasis on the exceptional durability, flexibility, and resistance to water damage that hemp fibers offer. These qualities made hemp rope an invaluable resource for various activities, such as construction, transportation, and maritime ventures. In the maritime context, for instance, hemp rope was less prone to rotting in damp conditions than ropes made from other materials available at the time.

The invention and application of tools derived from hemp are a testament to the innovative spirit and adaptability of past civilizations. Understanding the properties of hemp and transforming its fibers into durable, functional tools required knowledge, skills, and inventiveness. When placed in perspective, we should acknowledge how far humanity has progressed. Compared to today's technological advancements, even a simple achievement like the creation of durable rope marked a significant leap in the technological capabilities of societies. Consequently, the use of hemp throughout history provides insights into more than just archaeological artifacts. It speaks to the historical significance of the cannabis plant, its practical applications, and the ingenious ways early civilizations utilized its potential to advance collective development.

450–200 BC

The period from 450 to 200 BC marked an important period for the development of medical knowledge in the Greco-Roman world, with cannabis playing a significant role. Renowned physician Pedanius Dioscorides, who authored "De Materia Medica," an encyclopedia of medicinal plants, prescribed cannabis for ailments such as toothaches and earaches.

Around the same period, Greek physician Galen noted that cannabis was widely consumed throughout the Roman Empire. The plant was used not just as a medicine but also for recreational purposes, highlighting its widespread acceptance and incorporation into various facets of daily life. Women of the Roman elite were reported to have used cannabis to alleviate the pain of childbirth, another early acknowledgment of cannabis's pain-relieving properties.

Additionally, cannabis also continued to be recognized for its industrial value, with evidence of hemp rope usage in Greece. A testament to the growing understanding of the versatile uses of the plant in the European continent.

Furthermore, this era also witnessed the recognition of cannabis in the Chinese Book of Rites, where hemp fabric was mentioned. This significant Confucian text emphasizes the enduring and vital role that cannabis played in China for centuries before the Common Era. It's not shocking that China stands out as one of the very few countries that barely criminalized industrial hemp. Chinese hemp production, which is primarily for the fiber market, has been legal throughout most of China's history, as you may have noticed. However, hemp cultivation was banned in 1985, after China became part of the UN Convention on Psychotropic Substances (one of the International Drug Control Conventions), but as hemp stigmas lessened, China resumed production by 2010. The industry savvy country only made illegal high-THC cannabis and consumption. In the last twenty-four years China has evolved into the world's primary hemp supplier to date, while most other countries, including the US, adopted irrational policies that for the most part continue to be in effect today.

Perhaps, highly fascinating is the mentioning of cannabis in the history narratives written by Herodotus, one of the earliest document history experts in Europe. These important narratives describe and explain the long history of conflict between Greeks and non-Greeks, culminating in the Graeco-Persian Wars of the early fifth century. Herodotus references the Scythians' use of cannabis for recreational purposes.

100 BC

We are now in the year 100 BC. There is historical evidence that hemp continued to be a resource in China to produce paper, marking a significant milestone in the progression of human communication and record-keeping. In early civilizations, writing material was limited to clay tablets, papyrus rolls, and animal skins, each of which had significant limitations. Clay tablets were cumbersome and fragile, papyrus was expensive and not particularly durable, and animal skins required extensive processing.

Apparently, the invention of hemp paper revolutionized these practices. Made from the inner bark of the hemp plant, this new form of paper was both strong and versatile. The process of making hemp paper involved soaking the hemp fibers in water, pounding them into a pulp, and then setting the substance out to dry. The result was a flat, smooth surface ideal for writing.

This innovation notably streamlined the documentation and sharing of information, extending the durability and portability of written records. It also underscored hemps versatility, which was already renowned for its roles in textiles, rope production, medicinal purposes, and recreational use. During this era, when the plant was acknowledged for its various applications, it played a pivotal role in advancing communication and the exchange of knowledge. Cannabis, in tandem with the evolution of human civilization, consistently offered multifaceted utility to various facets of human existence.

0 AD

Well, there is no year 0; the calendar goes straight from 1 BC to 1 AD. But we can bet cannabis and hemp were present in the in-between time as well.

1 AD

The Bible was not written at a single point in time; rather, it is a compilation of texts that were written over many centuries. It is traditionally divided into two main sections: the Old Testament and the New Testament. The texts of the New Testament were written in Greek and are generally dated to the first century CE. They include the life and teachings of Jesus Christ, as well as the works and letters of his apostles. The earliest of these are the Pauline epistles, written between approximately 50 and 60 CE. The Gospels (Matthew, Mark, Luke, and John) were likely written between 70 and 100 CE.

One question that comes up frequently is whether cannabis is mentioned in the Bible or not. The Bible does not explicitly mention cannabis or hemp by that exact syntax. However, some researchers and religious scholars have suggested that certain herbs and plants mentioned in the Bible could be references to cannabis or hemp, but these interpretations are speculative and not universally accepted by Christians. One of the most cited examples is the term "kaneh-bosm" in the Hebrew Bible (Old Testament). This term appears in the book of Exodus and describes one of the ingredients in the holy anointing oil.

"Take the finest spices: of liquid myrrh five hundred shekels, and of sweet-smelling cinnamon half as much, that is, two hundred and fifty, and of <u>aromatic cane</u> two hundred and fifty. (Exodus 30:23, RSV)"

Some argue that "kaneh-bosm" could be a reference to cannabis, but the translation and interpretation are subject to debate, and there is no definitive evidence to support this claim. According to the Ancient Hebrew Research Center, the Hebrew phrase *qaneh bosem* can be defined as "an aromatic resinous reed plant" and may be descriptive of the cannabis plant. Ultimately, while there are numerous mentions of herbs, oils, and incense in the Bible, none can be definitively identified as cannabis or hemp. Hence, the Bible's stance on these plants remains a matter of interpretation, in the same fashion as many other matters found within its pages.

200–900 AD

Although the mention of cannabis in the Bible may be subject to speculation, there is solid historical evidence to prove that the use of cannabis for various purposes continued for thousands of years, weaving its roots across various cultures and civilizations. Research shows that during the period of 200 to 900 AD, the plant continued to see a range of applications, from medicinal to industrial, expanding its versatility and significance in many developing societies around the world.

Green Renaissance

Around 200 AD, the Eastern world's first pharmacopoeia listed medical cannabis, signifying an early recognition of the plant's therapeutic potential. Not long after, in 207 AD, Hua T'o, a Chinese physician, became the first known doctor to record cannabis as a sedative. He innovatively created a concoction of cannabis and wine to serve as a sedative for patients undergoing surgery... This is an interesting combination.

In the following century, around 300 AD, evidence emerged suggesting the use of cannabis during childbirth in Jerusalem. Another example of how the plant's pain-relieving properties were employed in women's health.

Meanwhile, the plant's industrial applications continued to sprout in Europe. By 500 AD, hemp began to be utilized for paper production in the European continent. In a testament to the quality and durability of hemp paper, it was even used to print bibles, marking an important milestone in the intersection of cannabis, religious history, and industrial development.

As the centuries rolled on, hemp's use expanded into the fashion industry. In 570 AD, Arnegunde, a French queen, was buried with hemp cloth, evidencing the material's prominence and value in elite society during the sixth century.

The cultivation of hemp received further attention in the sixth century, with the Confucian text "The Essential Arts for the People" (Qi Min Yao Shu) providing extensive coverage of the latest hemp cultivation techniques for the time. This ancient text is among the first to introduce the concepts of crop rotation and the use of potassium fertilizer, two techniques that continue to shape modern farming practices to this day.

The nineth century saw the advent of hemp's journey across the seas, with Vikings taking hemp rope and seeds to Iceland around 850 AD, showcasing the plant's practical utility and importance in seafaring expeditions during this era.

As the tenth century approached, circa 900 AD, historical records show the adoption of Arabian techniques in hemp paper production.

This event represents a significant exchange of technology, demonstrating the cross-cultural and cross-regional documentation of cannabis and hemp usage and processing methods.

The period between 200 and 900 AD stands out because of the multifaceted roles cannabis played in societies around the globe. The plant was woven into the fabric of cultures, playing important roles in significant advancements within major growing industries.

1000s–1900s

By this time, with the help of hemp paper, books, newspapers, and other print media were durable and portable, directly contributing to the documentation of our planet's history. Look at God! Based on the availability of information by this time, we can confirm that the use of cannabis throughout the period of 1000–1600 AD was varied and wide-ranging, extending across different cultures and geographical areas.

In the Middle East, cannabis continued to be used for its medicinal properties, particularly in the Islamic world. Islamic physicians considered cannabis a useful treatment for a variety of conditions, from migraines to fevers. The use of cannabis as a psychoactive substance was also known, although this was generally discouraged by religious authorities.

In Europe during the Middle Ages, hemp was primarily cultivated for its strong fibers. Hemp seeds were also used for their oil and as a food source. While the medicinal and psychoactive properties of cannabis were known in Europe at this time, the plant's use for these purposes had not yet become widespread.

During this time, in Italy, hemp was widely used in maritime ventures. Its strong fibers were crafted into ropes that were indispensable for Italian ships. The high tensile strength and durability of hemp-made ropes contributed to the successful voyages of Italian seafarers and traders.

In the East, cannabis also had a prominent role. In India, the use of cannabis for religious and medicinal purposes continued throughout this period. Cannabis was commonly consumed in a drink called bhang, which was used in religious ceremonies and as a medicinal preparation.

In China, the medicinal use of cannabis continued as well. Hemp continued to be used to treat a variety of conditions, including malaria, beriberi, constipation, rheumatic pains, absent-mindedness, and female disorders. Chinese doctors often used the seeds of the cannabis plant, known as "huo ma ren," rather than the flowers or leaves.

Arabic scholars had begun to identify and use cannabis as an effective treatment for epilepsy, a neurological disorder characterized by recurrent seizures. Al-Mayusi and al-Badri, two prominent scholars of the time, significantly contributed to this understanding. Their work provided an early foundation for the use of cannabis in treating epilepsy, a practice that is still being explored and validated by scientific research today. In a contrasting perspective, Arabic physician Ibn Wahshiyah cautioned against the potential dangers of marijuana in his seminal work, "On Poisons." His warnings were among the early acknowledgments of the potential negative effects of the substance, illustrating the long-standing debate about the benefits and risks of cannabis use. A debate many of us are very familiar with.

In Africa, the diverse uses of cannabis mirrored the multi-faceted understanding and engagement with the plant observed worldwide. Both in medicine and in social customs, cannabis was an integral part of various African societies.

As I mentioned earlier, in Egypt, the application of cannabis was well-documented. For instance, ancient Egyptian medicinal texts have referred to cannabis being used as a treatment for glaucoma. It is said that in Egypt, folks back then would take cannabis, grind it up with celery, and then let this concoction sit overnight. Once the sun came up, they'd use this unique mixture to rinse out the eyes of people who were dealing with glaucoma. These ancient Egyptian physicians recognized the anti-inflammatory properties of cannabis, using it as a topical treatment for eye conditions. Their pioneering use of cannabis in medicine contributes to the rich tapestry of the plant's historical medical applications.

Moving forward in our journey through history, we arrive at the 1300s. There's compelling proof in the form of smoking pipes from Ethiopia, which were found to contain remnants of cannabis. It's remarkable to think about how this humble plant managed to leave its imprint all around the world. This is another piece of the puzzle in understanding how deeply entwined the story of cannabis is with human evolution.

Elsewhere in Africa, cannabis was not only valued for its medical potential but also for its psychoactive effects. Its consumption was integrated into social and cultural rituals. For some communities, the use of cannabis in a recreational context was an embedded tradition, a part of communal gatherings or religious rituals. Showcasing the dichotomy in perceptions of cannabis that persist even today: a therapeutic substance and a recreational mood enhancer. Moreover, the plant was grown and harvested for other uses as well, including the production of textiles, rope, and other industrial materials.

For a long time, historical records indicated no presence of cannabis in the western hemisphere prior to its introduction by Spanish colonizers in 1545, primarily in the form of industrial hemp. An early documented mention of cannabis can be traced to South America, specifically in Chile's Quillota Valley. Here hemp cultivation thrived, primarily due to royal colonial mandates. Employing a mix of incentives and coercion, colonial authorities encouraged large landowners to engage in the cultivation of this indispensable fiber.

Moving northward, hemp held immense importance for the thirteen British colonies, where it was extensively grown for industrial purposes. However, although many reject any proof of hemp's presence in the New World prior to Christopher Columbus's arrival, there are historians who beg to differ. Their study indicates the findings of abundant examples of textile relics fashioned from hemp fiber. Could it be that pre-Columbian Indigenous peoples also engaged in the use of cannabis and hemp among tribes? It certainly seems like the probability is very likely! For the tribes, Hemp was primarily employed for crafting fabric, sandals, fishing nets, ropes, mats, and baskets, although it also played roles in rituals and medicine.

Hemp, being a dioecious plant, featuring distinct male and female genders, exhibits substantial genetic diversity, rendering it highly adaptable. Not to mention, the versatility of its uses makes an ideal species for colonizers to migrate with to new territories as a few seeds could go a long away.

Ethnologist W.H. Holmes, affiliated with the Smithsonian Institution, not only confirms the introduction of cannabis by the Vikings but also its presence in the New World during prehistoric times. He proposes that it was transported by both humans and animals across the Bering Strait, a strait between the Pacific and Arctic oceans, separating the Chukchi Peninsula of the Russian Far East from the Seward Peninsula of Alaska.

"The Vikings depended on hemp for their rope and sails, and they probably carried the seed with them and planted it when they visited North America about a thousand years ago. Sailors usually carried supplies of seeds with them to provide the necessities of life in the case of a shipwreck. Perhaps Christopher Columbus also did the good deed when he arrived in 1492, with the aid of over 80 tons of hemp rigging. Certainly, however, cannabis arrived in prehistoric times, possibly brought from China by explorers, and birds crossing the Bering Strait to the left coast of America." (Cyrus Gordon, *Before Columbus: Links Between the Old World & Ancient America*, 1971)

Indications of its existence are linked with the Mound Builders, pre-Columbian inhabitants of North America, whose history spans from 3,000 BCE to the sixteenth century CE. They resided in the Great Lakes and Mississippi River regions.

For rituals and textile production, they utilized cannabis, as evidenced by numerous pipes and sizable fabric remnants discovered.

Upon their passing, in addition to other grave items, spools of hemp thread used in crafting their textiles were buried alongside them.

As per historian Cyrus Gordon, when Christopher Columbus reached the New World, each of his vessels carried 180 tons of hemp rigging and sails. If cannabis had already grown in the New World during this era, it likely existed in limited areas and its utilization was significantly segmented throughout the population. Nevertheless, Spaniard conquistadors brought hemp (cáñamo) to New Spain, the territory we now know as Mexico in the sixteenth century. The hardy plant sprang up with the wind and scattered throughout the hills of Mexico's dry Sierras.

In 1524, Italian explorer Giovanni da Verrazzano first encountered wild cannabis during an expedition to Virginia in North America. French explorer Jacques Cartier reported vast expanses of wild cannabis on his voyages to what's now known as Canada between the years 1535 and 1541. Samuel de Champlain mentioned in 1605 that he observed natives employing wild hemp on their fishhooks. Nonetheless, hemp wasn't officially recognized as part of North America's flora until 1606.

In 1609, during his visit to Virginia with Thomas Hariot, Henry Spelman described how Indigenous people used hemp baskets to harvest maize. James Adair documented the Cherokee Indians and other tribes utilizing hemp in his book, *The History of the American Indians* (1775).

Throughout the million-year history of humanity, the hemp plant has played a pivotal role in aiding human survival, spreading across the world, and assisting us over countless millennia. We can expect continued progress in unraveling hemp's historical narrative, occasionally surprising us with our own past.

Navigating the seventeenth and eighteenth centuries, we see some fascinating developments in the story of cannabis. In the 1600s, England began importing hemp from Russia, setting the stage for the plant's cultivation on a much wider scale. Meanwhile, on the other side of the world, with colonization in full force, the Jamestown colonists in

America had also begun growing hemp by 1616, as the plant was essential to early settlers. As you can see, history has a tendency to repeat itself, with cannabis being deemed "essential" during the pandemic. More about that when we get to that time period.

America's founding fathers engaged in the cultivation of cannabis for various purposes, including industrial, medicinal, and occasional recreational use. George Washington and Thomas Jefferson, who had a distinct aversion to tobacco, are documented as having grown British hemp and even exchanged gifts of smoking blends. During the 1790s, Washington expanded his cultivation efforts to include "India Hemp," a resinous variety originating from India. During this period, cannabis went by multiple names, including "common hemp" (referring to C. sativa, cultivated for its fibers and seeds) and "India hemp" (pertaining to C. indica, cultivated for fibers and resin). It's essential to note that "India hemp" should not be confused with "Indian hemp" (Apocynum cannabinum, dogbane). In modern terms, "Indian hemp" refers to jute, an unrelated plant to *Cannabis Sativa*, and it was not introduced to America until a much later period.

Interestingly, America's first cannabis law was enacted in 1619 at Jamestown Colony, Virginia, not for prohibition purposes, but rather, to encourage all farmers to grow "India hemp" seed. A few years later, in 1621, Burton's Anatomy of Melancholy even suggested that the cannabis plant could potentially be used for depression therapy. The laws making hemp cultivation mandatory extended to Massachusetts in 1631 and Connecticut the following year.

It's worth mentioning that even across the pond in England, the Crown showed a keen interest in cannabis. Foreigners who grew the plant earned the highly coveted status of full British citizenship. Those who refused to cultivate hemp were often penalized with fines. Who would have known that cannabis would also be the solution to immigration issues? I'm just kidding! (But every joke has a grain of truth.)

The great Swedish botanist, Carl Linnaeus, classified the plant as Cannabis sativa in 1753. Carl Linnaeus made significant contributions to the field of botany, forever changing the way we classify and understand plant species. His most profound work was his system of binomial nomenclature, a method for naming organisms that is still in use today. This system consists of two parts: the genus and the species' name. In 1753, in his monumental work "Species Plantarum," Linnaeus applied this system to cannabis for the first time, giving it the scientific name "Cannabis sativa." The term "sativa" means "cultivated" in Latin, reflecting the plant's long history of cultivation by human societies.

The classification of the cannabis plant by Linnaeus was an essential step in the scientific understanding and study of this species. By providing it with a scientific name, Linnaeus gave researchers a common language to describe the plant, enabling more precise communication and study of its characteristics and effects.

In Linnaeus's time, Cannabis sativa was recognized mainly for its industrial uses, such as producing hemp fiber for rope, cloth, and paper. However, Linnaeus's classification paved the way for future scientific research into other aspects of the plant, including its medical and psychoactive properties. Despite Linnaeus's classification, the taxonomy of cannabis remains somewhat controversial, with debates about whether there are one, two, or three species within the genus Cannabis. Linnaeus identified the plant as a single species, Cannabis sativa.

The late eighteenth century was a significant period for both the agricultural and scientific understanding of cannabis. Across the Atlantic, two distinct events took place that would have enduring impacts on the trajectory of the plant's history.

In North America, the fertile soils of Kentucky quickly became recognized as prime lands for hemp cultivation. Amid the struggles of the American Revolution, Kentucky's initiative to delve into hemp cultivation was a timely decision. Hemp, a versatile and robust crop, was integral to the then young nation. It provided essential raw materials for indispensable items, including the paper on which the Declaration of Independence was written. Kentucky, with its agricultural propensity, was at the forefront of this movement. The Bluegrass

State's involvement in hemp cultivation would pave the way for it to become one of the leading hemp producers in the United States, a position it maintained for over a century.

In California, the introduction of Spanish hemp subsidies sparked an agricultural boom, resulting in the production of thousands of pounds of hemp annually from 1795 to 1810. However, as Mexico, which included California and most of the American Southwest, began to push for independence from the Spanish Crown, the royal subsidies vanished, causing the fledgling California hemp industry to wither away. Yet, the plant would reemerge, this time with a different purpose, during the mid-1800s gold rush. The gold rush drew a diverse influx of people from around the world, all seeking their fortunes in California's hills. In the foothills of the Golden State, various ethnic communities converged, each with its own unique historical relationships to cannabis and psychedelics.

By this time, cannabis was a medicinal staple in Mexico, and used recreationally for its calming properties. In the countryside, many citizens just self-medicated, using cannabis-centric recipes passed on down from family generations. Indigenous traditional healers also used cannabis as a medicinal herb.

While farmers from the New World were sowing their fields with hemp, across the ocean, the world of European botany was abuzz with the work of French naturalist Jean-Baptiste Lamarck. In 1783, Lamarck offered a new classification for the cannabis plant, naming it Cannabis indica. This was a departure from the earlier classification by the Swedish botanist Carl Linnaeus, who had identified the plant as Cannabis sativa in 1753. Lamarck's classification was based on the morphological differences he observed in cannabis plants from India. Unlike the taller, leaner Cannabis sativa plants, these were shorter and bushier. Beyond physical characteristics, the plants also differed in their psychoactive properties, with Cannabis indica often producing more sedative effects.

Lamarck's introduction of Cannabis indica illuminated the idea that there was more than one species or subspecies of cannabis. This revelation would profoundly influence subsequent research, breeding, and cultivation practices. His work underscored the diversity within the genus Cannabis and laid the foundation for ongoing debates about the taxonomy and characteristics of various cannabis strains.

These two events, though geographically distant, showcase the multifaceted history of cannabis. On one hand, there was the pragmatic and economic dimension represented by Kentucky's hemp cultivation. On the other, the meticulous and inquisitive world of European botany was deepening its understanding of the plant's taxonomy. Together, they paint a vivid picture of a period when cannabis was forging its path both as an agricultural mainstay and as a subject of scientific fascination.

The late eighteenth and early nineteenth centuries were also marked by significant developments in the medical and recreational use of the cannabis plant. The therapeutic properties of cannabis were documented in The New England Dispensatory in 1764. Such event carved a path for further exploration of the plant's medicinal potential to follow. The recognition of cannabis as a useful medicinal plant reached a new level when Irish doctor William O'Shaughnessy introduced its therapeutic uses to Western medicine in 1839. He found no negative medicinal effects, leading to a rapid rise in the plant's use in a pharmaceutical context. In 1842, O'Shaughnessy's research on cannabis was published in English medical journals, helping to spread knowledge about the plant's therapeutic potential. Around the same time, Napoleon's soldiers in Egypt discovered cannabis and hashish, bringing these substances back to France. This led to further scientific investigations into the plant's properties.

On the other hand, as early as 1846, in Mexico, references to cannabis were related to the military and not in a good way. Contrary to popular belief, according to renowned historian Isaac Campo, Mexican newspapers started the negative narrative against cannabis during these years, almost a century before the "reefer madness" in the United States. In his book, *Home Grown: Marihuana and the Origin of Mexico's War on Drugs*, the author conducts an analysis of nearly six hundred newspaper articles detailing the effects of "marijuana" reveals that the drug caused violence, madness, and crime from 1846 through 1920 becoming the first country to enact cannabis prohibition laws in the western hemisphere. Campo's book states that a worried news reporter published an article advising the public that Mexican troops had been struck down "by a strange sickness," adding that the men were "without strength, languid, confused, and often ended in a profound stupor." The reporter attributed the cause of such peculiar disorder to "marijuana, which the soldiers smoke as if it was tobacco."

In Campos's work, he points out that the narratives presented in American media were not novel but rather reflections of reports that had already surfaced in Mexican publications much earlier. He documents numerous incidents from before the turn of the twentieth century that share striking similarities: one describes a soldier who, under the influence of "marijuana', turned violent against his peers (as reported by El Monitor Republicano in 1878), another incident involves a soldier committing murder and wounding others after consuming cannabis (La Voz de México, 1888), and a case of a prisoner killing two inmates following marijuana use (El Pais, 1899).

Campos also provides insight into the possible etymology of the term "Marijuana," conjecturing an intriguing explanation. He elucidates that "Juan" was commonly used to represent the typical Mexican soldier, like the American usage of "Joe" and "Jane" for average individuals. The term for a soldier's companion, often referred to as Maria, combined with "Juan" to form "Maria-Juan," which likely evolved into "marijuana."

Club des Hashischins: A Bohemian Tale of nineteenth Century Paris

The mid-nineteenth century in Paris was an era of extraordinary intellectual and artistic development. It was a time when the worlds of art, literature, and science often mingled, fueled by a common curiosity about the mysteries of the human mind. At the heart of this intellectual fervor was a secretive society known as the Club des Hashischins (or Hashish Eaters Club), a gathering of artists, writers, and thinkers who explored altered states of consciousness through the consumption of hashish.

Operating between 1844 and 1849, the Club des Hashischins met at the Hôtel de Lauzun on the Île Saint-Louis, at the very heart of Paris. The club was inspired by tales of the Hashshashin, a medieval sect of Ismaili assassins in the Middle East who, as legend has it, consumed hashish. The founding members, most notably French psychiatrist Jacques-Joseph Moreau and writers Théophile Gautier and Charles Baudelaire, were intrigued by the mind-altering properties of hashish, which were still relatively unknown in Europe at the time.

To say that these meetings were a casual social gathering would be an understatement. Members were presented with a greenish paste made from a mixture of hashish, pistachios, cinnamon, cloves, and other ingredients. This concoction, referred to as "dawamesk," was ingested by club members in search of inspiration or a heightened sense of creativity. What followed were hours of vivid hallucinations, intellectual discoveries, and often pure hedonistic indulgence.

The club's pursuits weren't merely recreational. Jacques-Joseph Moreau was a pioneer in the study of psychotropic substances and their effects on the human psyche. He believed that hashish provided a pathway to understanding mental illnesses by inducing symptoms akin to those of conditions like schizophrenia or bipolar disorder. His book, *Du Hachisch et de l'Aliénation Mentale* (*Hashish and Mental Illness*), was one of the earliest scientific investigations into drug-induced states of mind.

However, not all members viewed hashish with unequivocal enthusiasm. Charles Baudelaire, one of France's most celebrated poets, had a complex relationship with the substance. Although initially fascinated by its effects, he eventually grew skeptical, believing that the artificial paradises induced by hashish and other substances could not replace natural inspiration. His work "Les Paradis Artificiels" ("Artificial

Paradises") reflects these conflicted views, offering a cautionary tale against the excessive use of substances for artistic or intellectual gains.

The Club des Hashischins was short-lived but left an indelible mark on the dialogue surrounding drug use, creativity, and the boundaries of human consciousness. Today, the Club serves as an evocative example of the complex relationship between society and psychoactive substances. As we grapple with questions surrounding the legalization, medicinal use, and societal impact of cannabis, it's worth looking back to this secretive Parisian society. They serve as a testament to the enduring human fascination with altered states: a quest for understanding that has both enlightened and perplexed us, from the salons of nineteenth-century Paris to the modern debates of the twenty-first century.

The rest of the nineteenth century saw cannabis gaining more recognition in both medical and recreational circles. It was included in the US Pharmacopoeia in 1851 and mentioned for recreational use in an American work by Whittier in 1854. By the turn of the twentieth century, medical cannabis was being used to treat a variety of conditions, from nausea and rheumatism to labor pain.

Evidently, the history of cannabis in the seventeenth, eighteenth, and nineteenth centuries paints a picture of a plant that played a crucial role in societies on both sides of the Atlantic. Its cultivation was not only encouraged but often required by law, showing how important this crop was to the economies of the time. The medical potential of cannabis was also increasingly recognized, leading to its inclusion in various pharmaceutical formulations and principal medical texts in many countries.

In tracing the historical trajectory of cannabis, we aim to provide a broader perspective for the ongoing discourse about its place in contemporary society. Our primary objective is to illustrate that cannabis, which currently remains a subject of considerable debate, has deep roots in our shared past. This history is woven with threads of utility, spirituality, industry, wellness, lifestyle, and culture. Although attempts have been made to tarnish, weaponize, and obscure this historical tapestry for political reasons, its relevance persists.

Green Renaissance is a personal invitation for you to join me on this voyage of rediscovery, to understand why this plant has exerted such a profound influence on human history, and why its full potential cannot be disregarded. I encourage you to approach this narrative with an open mind, as it is only through such openness that we can fully grasp the intricate interplay between humanity and this remarkable plant.

Ultimately, this is not solely about the history of a plant; it is a narrative about humanity, evolution, and our intricate relationship with the natural world.

Chapter 3
The Beginning of Prohibition

The narrative of cannabis, a plant once revered for its multitude of uses, both therapeutic and industrial, began to shift dramatically during the twentieth century. Historically celebrated and integrated into numerous cultures worldwide, the perception of cannabis underwent a transformation that would alter its course for decades to come. But what factors precipitated this change? How did a plant, once considered indispensable, become the target of stringent regulations, negative propaganda, and widespread demonization?

The journey from widespread acceptance to prohibition is full of political, cultural, and economic agendas. By the end of this exploration, I hope to have discovered a better understanding of how cannabis, a plant with such deep historical roots in human civilization, became one of the most controversial and debated topics in modern history. It's a story that encompasses more than just the plant itself. It's about the very nature of societal control, the power of narratives, and the consequences of misinformation. As we spill the tea, we'll uncover the motives, agendas, and fears that accelerated cannabis's descent from a cherished crop to outlawed.

1908: King of the Grifos *[Stoners]*

Mexico City, Mexico, is home to one of the first cannabis arrests. José del Moral, dubbed as the King of the grifos and Mexico's City's poisoner in chief, was arrested at his home in Mexico. The fifty-year-old man was the Mexican capital's biggest cannabis wholesaler. A few days prior to his arrest, the Mexican police raided his warehouse, where they found thousands of cannabis cigarettes. He was sentenced to five months in prison and his crime: selling marijuana illegally. *El Imparcial,* a respected newspaper at the time, reacted with full-blown hysteria, making reference to del Moral's operations as a Marijuana Factory with enough product to "poison the entire population of Mexico City." Another news and media outlet, *El País,* referred to cannabis at the time as "the terrible cannabis indica of the healers is now the opium of our lower classes."

José del Moral might have also been one of the first documented cannabis activists. While serving his mandated sentence at Belén Prison, he wrote a very eloquent appeal letter:

> *"Doctors have denounced marijuana with limited knowledge about it. They don't make any mentions of studies and ignore the everyday applications of the herb. Instead, they simply chose to adopt the growing prejudices of those who run when they hear its very name and believe it has come from hell; and parrot the tabloids making up tales of marijuana-induced madness and weed-fueled murders. How can marijuana be considered dangerous for health... when it is used as a medicine for infinite ailments?"* (José del Moral, 1908)

Oddly enough, two years after José del Moral's imprisonment, the outbreak of the Mexican Revolution would drive thousands of Mexicans to cannabis consumption as a medicine as well as a relaxant; becoming the drug of choice for soldiers. Toward the end of the nineteenth century, cannabis medical and recreational consumption became minimal within Mexico's society. The plant was contained to tiny corner of Indigenous healers' stands, the military barracks, and prisons' walls. After the Revolution, it would remain as the drug of choice for bohemians and the lower class.

If you are business minded like me, you may be asking yourself, who was del Moral's ideal customer back then. In Mexican towns and cities, wholesalers like José del Moral sold cannabis to traditional healers also known as *herbolarias*. Herbolarias were Indigenous women who sold their advice and a myriad of herbs, barks, remedies, and potions at the country's hundreds of markets. Cannabis was one of their most versatile remedies. At the time, it was rolled up and smoked to treat bronchitis, asthma, and other respiratory conditions; it was applied as a topical in the form of powder or oil and rubbed on the stomachs of birthing women, rheumatic joints, and other physical pain ailments. Furthermore, it was dissolved in water combined with jimson weed and butter to make a "calming ointment" and boiled in water to produce a form of hash meant to be mixed with cinnamon syrup.

1913 California, Who Would Have Thought?!

Given its ties and proximity to Mexico, which had already engaged in cannabis criminalization, it is not surprising that California originated cannabis prohibition. In 1913, the state of California was the first state to start the prohibition crusade in the United States, a move instigated by the state's Board of Pharmacy as part of a broader, assertive campaign against narcotics, initially targeted at opiates. At that time, there was no widespread public concern regarding cannabis. The historical evidence for the use of "hashish" in California prior to 1913 is notably scarce. Historical evidence indicates that the term "Mexican marihuana" did not gain public familiarity until after the law's enactment.

Notably, the law's original proponent was board member Henry Finger, who allegedly advocated for it to prevent the proliferation of cannabis use among "Hindoo" immigrants. In 1914, the board-initiated raids against marihuana in the Mexican community of Los Angeles.

Despite the implementation of increasingly stringent penalties, cannabis use gradually expanded during the 1920s and beyond. It's important to emphasize that all of this was happening in California before "reefer madness," and was not originated due to a publicly perceived crisis about cannabis usage, but rather by a proactive bureaucratic endeavor on behalf of a state organization.

Harrison Narcotics Tax Act in 1914

The demonization of cannabis may have been cemented into the American fabric through a pivotal piece of legislation that set the tone for drug control in the United States: The Harrison Narcotics Tax Act of 1914. This act marked the beginning of the nation's long journey into prohibition, setting in motion a series of legislative actions that would culminate in the outright criminalization of many substances, including cannabis.

The Harrison Narcotics Tax Act wasn't just a law; it was a reflection of the growing anxieties of the early twentieth century. America was changing rapidly, with urban areas booming and societal norms being questioned. Amid this backdrop, psychoactive substances like opium and cocaine, once seen as medicinal wonders (believe it or not), were increasingly perceived as threats, especially in the hands of certain communities.

The act itself was primarily aimed at curbing the opioid epidemic of the time, placing strict regulations on the production and distribution of opiates and coca-derived products. Cannabis, while mentioned, wasn't the primary focus. However, the penalties set by the act were rather stringent. Traffickers could face fines of up to $50,000 or imprisonment of up to five years, depending on the severity of the crime and the amount of drugs confiscated.

The act had a very peculiar stance on cannabis. While selling heroin without a prescription from one's home was clearly criminalized, the sale of cannabis from one's home took on a murkier position. If a person was found selling cannabis in a space where heroin was sold without a prescription, the penalties mirrored those of selling heroin. However, the sale of cannabis on its own wasn't directly targeted by the act. This could be seen as a precursor to the governmental ambivalence that would later envelop cannabis in a cloud of misinformation and fear.

Fast forward to 1936, a mere two decades later, and the perception of cannabis had dramatically shifted. By this time, the Narcotic Bureau of the New York Police Department seized and destroyed a staggering 40,000 pounds of cannabis plants found within the city limits. Reflecting its increasing demand, cannabis was priced exorbitantly, reaching upward of $60 a pound at the time. This price points out the plant's significant presence in the recreational and, perhaps, medicinal landscape in America during the 1930s.

By this time, the tides were turning. The once-beloved cannabis plant was now in the crosshairs of regulatory bodies and public opinion.

Marihuana Tax Act of 1937

The late 1930s bore witness to an important turn of events in America's stance on cannabis. The Marihuana Tax Act of 1937 serves as a landmark in the history of cannabis regulation, presenting a unique conundrum. While it didn't outright criminalize the use or sale of cannabis, its implementation set a precedent that would echo throughout history, effectively choking the once-thriving commercialization of the plant as a commodity.

In a land where vast stretches of hemp fields were once common, the notion of criminalizing this versatile plant would have been inconceivable to earlier generations. Before the act, cannabis grew freely, an agricultural staple woven into the very fabric of America's farming community. Yet, with the stroke of a pen, this flourishing scene was set to change dramatically.

The Marihuana Tax Act wasn't solely about imposing a fee on the growth, sale, or import of cannabis, though that was a significant facet of it. The act symbolized a transition, marking cannabis as a substance to be controlled and stigmatized.

The legislation was rapidly embraced, passing through the House in 1938, and subsequently receiving President Franklin Delano Roosevelt's seal of approval. However, its rapid enforcement caught many off-guard. A mere three days after the act went into effect, Samuel R. Caldwell and Moses Baca found themselves entangled by the new law at Denver's Lexington Hotel. Their crime? A transaction that involved a mere two joints. Such immediate and severe action demonstrated the newfound seriousness with which the US government approached cannabis immediately after the Tax Act went live.

Yet, to understand the true motivations behind the act, we must look deeper, beyond the legal texts and into the social structure of the era. The 1930s was a tumultuous decade, with extensive racial tensions. Cannabis consumption, associated predominantly with Black Americans and Mexican immigrants, was frequently portrayed in a negative light, with the media and officials stoking fears and peddling misinformation. This racial underpinning is believed to have influenced the act's inception. Was the tax a covert tool of racial control? While opinions vary, there's no doubt that it disproportionately impacted Black and Brown communities.

Moreover, the tax itself was more than just a financial burden; it became a scarlet letter for those involved in the cannabis trade. The requirement to pay the tax was equivalent to self-incrimination for many OG canna-preneurs. In an era where being associated with cannabis could get you jail time, many chose to forgo the tax, diving into the shadows and operating beyond the reach of the law. This reluctance to comply sowed the seeds for the next phase in America's complex relationship with cannabis and the birth of the so-called black market.

Reefer Madness Origins

The passage of the Marihuana Tax Act of 1937 ushered in what is often referred to as the "Darkest Period" in the history of cannabis in the United States. Spanning from 1937 into the 1960s, this era was punctuated by a cascade of propaganda, misinformation, and intense persecution against cannabis and cannabis consumers. But what made this time especially vexing was that this was the point of no return from the departure from a previous era, where cannabis and hemp were cultivated and utilized for their many beneficial purposes.

During these dark decades, the flames of "reefer madness" were fervently fanned. A lurid tapestry of falsehoods was painted, where the once considered beneficial cannabis plant was now the villain in a drama that the government and media eagerly perpetuated. Gone were the days when the plant was seen as a medical remedy; instead, a sinister narrative was promoted, depicting cannabis as a dangerous drug threatening to corrupt the moral fabric of society. Complicit in this widespread demonization were major media outlets that voraciously consumed and regurgitated the anti-cannabis narrative with headlines and stories often sensationalizing accounts of crimes allegedly committed under its influence, instilling fear and apprehension in the public mind.

These campaigns of misinformation weren't limited to the media. Even governmental bodies, which the public inherently trusted for impartial information, played their part in perpetuating the myths. The Department of Agriculture, in an unexpected departure from its typical mandate, launched a concerted smear campaign. Their portrayal of cannabis users was far from flattering, painting them as violent, deranged, and morally bankrupt individuals.

It was against this widespread misinformation and public paranoia that Samuel R. Caldwell found himself ensnared by the law. As the first person to be arrested for cannabis possession post the Tax Act, his arrest wasn't just a legal event—it was symbolic. It sent a clear message: the era of tolerance for cannabis had come to an end. The subsequent media coverage and public discourse surrounding Caldwell's arrest underscored the deep divisions and contentious debates the topic of cannabis had ignited across the nation.

To say that the country was divided would be an understatement. On one side, there were those who, fueled by propaganda, viewed cannabis and cannabis consumers as a menace to society. On the other, a marginalized group argued for its medicinal properties and the rights of individuals to choose. This chasm between the two perspectives only deepened as the years wore on, setting the stage for future battles over cannabis, legalization, criminalization, and its place in society.

1942: Hemp for Victory: America's Wartime Paradox

The year was 1942, and America found itself in the throes of World War II, a conflict that would redefine global society and national interests. Amid the chaos, an unforeseen problem emerged: a dire shortage of hemp, a crop essential for making ropes, parachutes, and other wartime necessities. The war had cut off access to key international suppliers, forcing the US government to look inward. What followed was a striking about-face in policy, the "Hemp for Victory" campaign, an initiative that flies in the face of modern perceptions of cannabis and reveals a contradictory, complex relationship between America and the versatile plant.

At the heart of "Hemp for Victory" was a full-blown, government-sanctioned push for the re- cultivation of hemp, which by then was already known to be a variety of the "frowned upon" cannabis plant. Farmers were encouraged to plant it as part of their patriotic duty to the nation. The US Department of Agriculture even produced an instructional film of the same name to educate the public and rally them around hemp cultivation. This monumental effort resulted in over 400,000 acres of hemp being planted and harvested, effectively reviving a then-dying industry. It's an irony that can't be understated: this very government would later go to great lengths to criminalize all forms of cannabis, citing it as a societal ill.

The paradox of the "Hemp for Victory" campaign can be seen as a powerful testament to the many uses of cannabis that stretch far beyond its psychoactive properties. While much of today's conversation around cannabis legalization focuses on its medicinal or recreational uses, the "Hemp for Victory" campaign highlights an often overlooked yet crucial aspect of *Cannabis sativa L* a.k.a. hemp—its utility as an industrial resource. Whether for textiles, paper, or biofuel, hemp provides a sustainable, eco-friendly alternative to many other materials.

"Long ago, when these ancient Grecian temples were new, hemp was already old in the service of humankind. For thousands of years, even then, this plant had been grown for cordage and cloth in China and elsewhere in the East. For centuries prior to about 1850, all the ships that sailed the western seas were rigged with hempen rope and sails. For the sailor, no less than the hangman, hemp was indispensable." ("Hemp for Victory" transcript, 1942)

The campaign not only challenges preconceptions about cannabis but also serves as a lens for examining the changeability of public policy. The US government didn't just tolerate hemp during this period; it actively promoted its cultivation, creating an infrastructure that saw it as a critical national resource. This chapter in cannabis history underscores the need for a nuanced, evidence-based approach to cannabis policy, revealing that views and laws can shift dramatically when national interests are at stake.

The end of World War II saw the phasing out of the "Hemp for Victory" program, but its implications linger on. With a modern backdrop of increasingly liberal state laws but continued federal prohibition, this campaign forces us to question the inconsistencies and contradictions in the United States' relationship with cannabis. It challenges the stigma, inviting us to consider the plant not just as a medicinal miracle or recreational delight, but as a multi-faceted asset that has played various roles throughout history.

So, as we grapple with the future of cannabis—navigating legal landscapes, dissecting medical research, and confronting societal norms —let us remember this unique era. "Hemp For Victory" serves not merely as a wartime anecdote but as a compelling case for reevaluating the role of cannabis in America. This seemingly forgotten campaign reminds us that attitudes can change, stigmas can be broken, and what was once considered invaluable can be cast aside—all due to the fluctuating tides of societal perception and need. It is a lesson in the malleability of public sentiment and policy, offering a glimpse into what could be possible for cannabis once again.

1960: Raphael Mechoulam and the Pioneering Discovery of THC

The story of cannabis and its complex relationship with humanity took a sharp turn in the mid-twentieth century. This pivot came about, not because of any policy change or societal shift, but due to groundbreaking scientific research. Central to this narrative was the work of an Israeli chemist named Raphael Mechoulam. His research in the 1960s would forever alter our understanding of cannabis, setting the stage for decades of scientific inquiry.

By the early 1960s, the chemistry of cannabis remained an enigma. While the plant's psychoactive properties were well known, mainly due to anecdotal experiences, the specific molecule responsible for this effect had eluded discovery. That changed in 1964 when Professor Raphael Mechoulam, working at the Hebrew University of Jerusalem, successfully isolated and synthesized the molecule delta9-tetrahydrocannabinol, commonly known as THC. This was the first time the primary psychoactive component of cannabis had been isolated in its pure form.

The implications of Mechoulam's work were profound. With the isolation of THC, scientists could now study the molecule's effects on the human body in isolation, paving the way for a deeper understanding of how cannabis interacts with the human brain and body. The paper titled "Isolation, structure and partial synthesis of an active constituent of hashish," published in the prestigious Journal of the American Chemical Society, stands testament to this defining moment in cannabinoid research.

But Mechoulam's curiosity about cannabis did not stop with THC. Recognizing the plant's rich chemical composition, he and his team pressed ahead, undertaking the synthesis of other major cannabinoids, such as cannabidiol (CBD) and cannabigerol (CBG). Each of these compounds, like THC, possesses unique properties and potential therapeutic applications.

Yet, perhaps the most fascinating twist in Mechoulam's storied career came with the discovery of endocannabinoids. These are naturally occurring compounds in the human body that mimic the actions of cannabinoids. The most notable of these, anandamide, was isolated and characterized by Lumír Ondřej Hanuš and William Devane, two researchers working under Mechoulam. Anandamide, named after the Sanskrit word "ananda" meaning "bliss," was the first endocannabinoid to be identified. The subsequent discovery of 2-AG, another endocannabinoid, by Shimon Ben-Shabat, a doctoral student of Mechoulam's, added yet another layer to the complex interplay between cannabinoids and human biology.

Over a career spanning decades and with more than 350 scientific articles to his name, Raphael Mechoulam has rightfully earned his reputation as "the father of cannabis research." His work laid the foundation for understanding not only the plant's pharmacology but also its potential therapeutic benefits. In a world where cannabis policy is rapidly evolving, the pioneering work of Mechoulam and his team serves as a reminder of the importance of science in guiding our understanding and approach to this ancient plant.

The Mecca of American Cannabis Cultivation

The Emerald Triangle, comprising Humboldt, Mendocino, and Trinity counties in Northern California, has long been considered the Mecca of cannabis cultivation. This region has gained near-mythic status among both the canna-curious and connoisseurs, largely due to the quality and quantity of cannabis it produces. The area's unique microclimates, rich soil, and generations of cultivation know-how make it particularly well-suited for cannabis farming.

Emerging in the late 1960s and solidifying its reputation through the 1970s and 1980s, the Emerald Triangle became a haven for countercultural individuals, including Vietnam War veterans and back-to-the-landers who sought a simpler, off-grid lifestyle. The remote, forested landscape offered an ideal setting for covert cannabis farming, especially during the years of cannabis prohibition. Many of these pioneers had a deep respect for the land and practiced sustainable farming methods long before such concepts were mainstream.

As laws began to change, especially with California's Proposition 215 in 1996, which legalized medical marijuana, and later with Proposition 64 in 2016, which legalized recreational use, the Emerald Triangle started transitioning from an underground operation to a more mainstream, though still iconic, part of American industry. Yet, it's not just the volume or legality that makes the Triangle iconic; it's also the community of growers who treat cannabis cultivation as both an art and a science. The region has produced some of the most celebrated strains in the world, many of which have won prestigious awards.

However, the area is not without its challenges. The increased commercialization of cannabis has brought with it a host of issues, including environmental concerns like illegal water diversion, pesticide use, and deforestation. Additionally, the influx of large-scale commercial operations threatens to edge out the smaller, independent farmers who have been the backbone of the Emerald Triangle for several decades. Despite these challenges, the Emerald Triangle remains a symbol of high-quality, artisanal cannabis cultivation.

I had the pleasure to meet Doc Ray, a true pioneer and veteran in the world of cannabis hailing out of the Emerald Triangle, in 2020. He stands as a testament to the incredible journey this plant has taken from its clandestine origins to becoming a source of healing and hope for many. With over five decades of working in many aspects of the plant dating back to 1972, he has witnessed and contributed to the evolution of medicinal cannabis from the shadows into the forefront of plant medicine.

His journey as a Cannabis Breeder and Cultivator has been marked by unwavering dedication. Since 1984, he's been a Pheno-Specific Cannabis Chemovar Breeder, a path that led him to join the esteemed Mendocino Green Mountain Growers group. But Doc's relationship with cannabis is far more than professional; it's deeply personal. As an Army Green Beret, he discovered the therapeutic potential of cannabis in the 1970s while grappling with the physical and emotional toll of his military service. This experience sparked a lifelong mission to explore the healing properties of this remarkable plant, not just for himself but for the entire veteran community.

Over the years, Doc Ray has delved into every conceivable method of cannabis cultivation, from full sun to indoor environments. His preferred methodology involves indoor HP Aeroponic Co2 enhanced techniques and sun-grown custom-blended organic living soil. But it's not just about growing; it's about healing. For the past three decades, he's been at the forefront of the medical cannabis movement. He's helped patients with a wide array of conditions, from childhood epilepsy to various forms of cancer, severe physical injuries, and even emotional and mental health challenges. Over the years, I've learned that Doc's commitment to cannabis as a tool for wellness knows no bounds, and he's continued to push the boundaries of what this plant can offer.

A Paradigm Shift: The 1970s and The Controlled Substances Act

The 1970s was a tumultuous decade, marked by the Vietnam War, the civil rights movement, and sweeping social change. Amid this complex social environment, the US government took a decisive stance against drug use with the enactment of the Controlled Substances Act (CSA) in 1970. This legislation would come to be one of the most influential and controversial drug laws in the nation's history, profoundly reshaping the country's attitude toward drugs and drug use.

One of the most contentious aspects of the CSA was its categorization of cannabis as a Schedule I substance. This classification placed cannabis in the most restrictive category alongside drugs such as heroin. By definition, Schedule I substances were believed to possess a high potential for abuse, offer no recognized medical use, and lack safety for use even under medical supervision. This classification was particularly alarming given the millennia-old history of cannabis as a medicinal plant, as well as the growing body of research suggesting its therapeutic potential.

However, the CSA didn't merely classify substances; it established the architecture for federal drug policy enforcement. The creation of the Drug Enforcement Administration (DEA) was a pivotal move stemming from the CSA. This agency, vested with broad powers and resources, was mandated to combat drug trafficking and abuse on both domestic and international fronts.

With cannabis now firmly in the crosshairs as a controlled substance, the DEA's intervention became relentless. Its classification meant that cultivation, distribution, and possession were illegal under federal law. DEA agents, armed with this mandate, launched aggressive campaigns against cannabis growers and suppliers, irrespective of the scale of their operations. Families growing a few plants for personal use were subjected to the same scrutiny as larger, commercial-scale operations. The law, with its unforgiving and extreme nature, showed no distinction between individual users and major traffickers.

The fallout of the CSA was multifaceted. On the one hand, it set the tone for decades of drug policy in the US, leading to the incarceration of millions for nonviolent drug offenses. On the other, it catalyzed a burgeoning underground market for cannabis, driving its trade into the shadows and bolstering organized crime networks. This climate of suppression and criminalization created a rift between law enforcement and communities, setting the stage for future debates and reforms.

Here's a brief overview of the Controlled Substances Act classification:

- *Schedule I*: Substances in this category are considered to have a high potential for abuse, no currently accepted medical use, and a lack of accepted safety for use under medical supervision. Examples include heroin, LSD, and, controversially, cannabis.
- *Schedule II*: These substances also have a high potential for abuse but also have some accepted medical uses with severe restrictions. Abuse of these substances may lead to severe physical or psychological dependence. Examples include cocaine, methamphetamine, and powerful opioids like oxycodone and fentanyl.
- *Schedule III*: Substances in this category are considered to have a moderate to low potential for physical and psychological dependence. They have accepted medical uses and include products with less than ninety milligrams of codeine, steroids, and ketamine.
- *Schedule IV*: These substances have a low potential for abuse relative to substances in Schedule III and include items like Xanax, Soma, and Valium. They are generally used for treating anxiety, panic attacks, and various other forms of neuroses.
- *Schedule V*: This is the least restrictive category and includes substances that have a lower potential for abuse than Schedule IV substances and contain limited amounts of certain narcotics. These are often used for antidiarrheal, antitussive, and analgesic purposes. Examples include cough preparations with less than 200 milligrams of codeine per 100 milliliters or per 100 grams.

The scheduling system has been the subject of controversy and calls for reform, particularly around the classification of cannabis as a

Schedule I drug, despite increasing evidence of its medical utility and widespread efforts at state-level legalization.

In hindsight, while the Controlled Substances Act of 1970 was designed with the intent of "protecting society" from the perceived dangers of drug abuse, it inadvertently sowed the seeds for many of the challenges the nation would face in the subsequent decades. The path to reevaluating and reshaping the legal landscape around cannabis had only just begun.

A Ruthless Turn: Rockefeller Drug Laws

The late 1970s marked a period of intensifying drug hysteria in the United States. As a reflection of this sentiment, a suite of notoriously stringent drug laws was passed in New York, which would soon set a precedent for the entire nation. Named after Governor Nelson Rockefeller, who fervently pushed for their enactment, the Rockefeller Drug Laws took America's already rigorous drug policies and supercharged them, ushering in an era of severe penalties for drug offenses.

The intent behind the Rockefeller Drug Laws was simple: eradicate drug-related crimes by implementing mandatory minimum sentences for those involved in the drug trade. On the surface, this strategy seemed straightforward enough—by removing drug offenders from the streets, the state could theoretically dismantle the drug trade piece by piece. However, the practical implications of this approach were far more complex and laden with unintended consequences.

Under the Rockefeller Drug Laws, even minor drug offenses were treated with unprecedented severity. Someone found in possession of a small quantity of a controlled substance, including cannabis, could face a minimum of fifteen years in prison. To provide context, these penalties were on par with those handed down for crimes like rape or manslaughter. The glaring disparity between the nature of the crime and the punishment it garnered was a subject of intense debate.

Contrary to its intention of curbing drug-related crimes, the Rockefeller Drug Laws resulted in a series of troubling outcomes. The state's prison population ballooned, straining the criminal justice system to this day. Many of these incarcerated individuals were nonviolent offenders caught with small amounts of drugs. Instead of focusing on rehabilitation or addressing the root causes of drug addiction, the state chose punitive incarceration, perpetuating a cycle of recidivism.

Moreover, these laws disproportionately affected Black and Brown communities, particularly African Americans and Hispanics, leading to widespread allegations of racial bias. This racial disproportion in arrests and convictions deepened the rift between law enforcement agencies and the communities they served, sowing seeds of distrust and resentment that carry on to this day in the US.

The backlash against the Rockefeller Drug Laws was substantial. Advocacy groups, legal experts, and even some law enforcement officials began calling for their repeal or significant amendment, citing the devastating social and economic consequences they had ushered in. The 1970s, a decade marked by counterculture movements and growing skepticism toward establishment views, also witnessed the foundation of critical organizations in the cannabis movement. High Times magazine and the National Organization for the Reform of Marijuana Laws (NORML) were both established during this era, amplifying the voices that advocated for cannabis reform and providing resources and information to those who needed it most. More on these organizations and the roles they played in a later chapter.

Over time, recognizing the myriad issues stemming from these laws, New York began to roll back some of its harshest provisions. By the early twenty-first century, there was a marked shift toward a more rehabilitative and less punitive approach to drug offenses, acknowledging that the "War on Drugs" strategy, epitomized by the Rockefeller Drug Laws, had largely failed. Today, the Rockefeller Drug Laws stand as a cautionary tale—a stark reminder of the perils of policy decisions guided by fear rather than evidence, and of the profound and lasting impacts such decisions can have on society. More on this evolution when we get to discussing the twenty-first century.

1985 Foundations of the Modern Hemp Movement

Jack Herer, often dubbed "the Emperor of Hemp," was not just an author but a fervent activist who dedicated a significant portion of his life to advocating for the cannabis plant. His book, *The Emperor Wears No Clothes*, published in 1985, is often considered the foundational text for the modern hemp movement.

The book meticulously breaks down the rich history of hemp as a versatile agricultural commodity. Herer dives deep into hemp's wide-ranging applications, from its uses in making durable textiles, paper, and building materials to its potential as a sustainable biofuel source. Additionally, he highlights the plant's nutritional benefits when consumed as food and its numerous therapeutic properties as a medicine.

What makes the book truly revolutionary is its exposé on the deliberate marginalization and demonization of cannabis, primarily driven by industrial interests in the early twentieth century. Herer posits that the prohibition of cannabis was less about its psychoactive properties and more about the threat it posed to established industries like timber, petroleum, and synthetic textiles. One of the book's main contentions is the way it lays out the economic incentives behind cannabis prohibition, detailing the involvement of influential figures like William Randolph Hearst and the Dupont family, who, Herer claims, had vested interests in sidelining hemp to protect their businesses.

Beyond just being a historical exposé, *The Emperor Wears No Clothes* was a call to action. Herer passionately argued for the decriminalization and full legalization of cannabis, seeing it as a path to environmental sustainability, economic revitalization, and an end to the unjust criminalization of its users. He believed that reintroducing hemp into the American agricultural and industrial landscapes could be a solution to many ecological and economic issues. The book's influence cannot be overstated. It galvanized a new generation of cannabis activists and informed public debate on the topic. Many of the arguments that are now commonly made about the benefits of cannabis and hemp can be traced back to Herer's work.

Jack Herer's enduring legacy is a testament to the power of well-researched advocacy. As discussions about sustainability and green solutions become more mainstream, the insights offered in *The Emperor Wears No Clothes* seem more pertinent than ever. The effects of climate change are becoming increasingly evident, underscoring the urgent need for sustainable solutions. Herer's insights and advocacy, which emphasized hemp's potential as an ecological panacea, appear even more prophetic now. As more countries and states move toward cannabis legalization, both for medical and recreational use, they're also discovering the vast industrial potential of hemp.

The current shift toward recognizing this potential is a testament to the tireless efforts of activists like Herer, whose groundbreaking work laid the foundation for the modern hemp revolution. Today, as industries pivot toward more sustainable practices and consumers demand eco-friendly products, the teachings from *The Emperor Wears No Clothes* offer invaluable guidance. Herer's work is the very inspiration for this book, as I truly believe that the future Jack Herer envisioned may be closer than we think.

1988: Dawn of the Endocannabinoid System

While the authorities ramped up the criminalization of cannabis, scientists were tirelessly searching for information about how this plant interacts with the human body. Their curiosity and dedication would soon bear fruit in 1988 with a groundbreaking discovery that would deepen our understanding of human biology and the psychoactive effects of cannabis. For many years, the scientific community had been puzzled: how could a plant like cannabis have such a profound and varied impact on the human body and mind? The answer began to take shape with the discovery of the CB1 and CB2 cannabinoid receptors, critical components of what we now recognize as the endocannabinoid system.

At the St. Louis University School of Medicine, Allyn Howlett and William Devane located the first of these receptors, CB1, within the brain. This revelation was monumental, offering the first concrete evidence of a biochemical mechanism through which cannabinoids, like THC, directly interact with the brain. CB1 receptors, primarily found in the brain and central nervous system, play a significant role in physiological processes, including mood regulation, appetite stimulation, and pain perception.

Following the unveiling of CB1 receptors, the CB2 receptors were soon identified. These receptors, in contrast to CB1, are mainly located in the peripheral organs, especially cells associated with the immune system, playing pivotal roles in mediating anti-inflammatory effects and other immune responses. One of the most striking revelations was the sheer abundance of CB1 receptors in the brain. They are among the most plentiful neuroreceptors present, rivaling even the density of major neurotransmitter receptors.

Beyond just explaining how cannabis compounds interacted with the human body, the discovery of these receptors set the stage for the identification of endocannabinoids. These naturally occurring molecules in our bodies, like anandamide and 2-AG, engage with these receptors, playing an essential role in maintaining physiological balance or homeostasis.

Understanding the endocannabinoid system was transformative. Not only did it provide insights into the effects of cannabis, but it also presented new avenues for medical research and therapeutic uses. Harnessing the potential of the endocannabinoid system to address conditions ranging from chronic pain to epilepsy, and even psychiatric disorders, has become one of the most exciting frontiers in medical research.

1992 San Francisco Cannabis Buyers Club: A Beacon of Hope and Resistance

Amid a dire AIDS epidemic and the accompanying pain and suffering that affected countless individuals in the 1990s, the San Francisco Cannabis Buyers Club emerged as a beacon of hope. Not just a simple dispensary, it was a grassroots effort that stood as a testament to community resilience, compassion, and activism against the heavy backdrop of cannabis criminalization.

The San Francisco Cannabis Buyers Club was founded in 1992 by Dennis Peron, a Vietnam War veteran and cannabis rights activist. Following the tragic loss of his partner to AIDS, Peron recognized the immense therapeutic benefits that cannabis could provide to those suffering from the disease. In an act of defiance against the establishment and with a spirit of compassion, he decided to open the club as a safe space where AIDS patients could purchase and use cannabis without the looming threat of law enforcement.

Operating out of a multi-story building in the heart of San Francisco, the club was not a typical "store." Beyond selling cannabis, it created a community environment where patients, many of whom were marginalized or ostracized because of their illness, could gather, support each other, and share their experiences. The environment was deliberately designed to be homey and welcoming, with couches, art, and even an on-site café. Educational sessions about the various strains of cannabis, methods of consumption, and the potential benefits and side effects were regularly conducted. This was crucial at a time when reliable information on medical cannabis was scarce, and most physicians were hesitant to recommend it.

The San Francisco Cannabis Buyers Club quickly grew to have a membership in the thousands, serving not only AIDS patients but also individuals with cancer, glaucoma, and other debilitating conditions. It was a revolutionary establishment in California's pre-Proposition 215 era, operating in a legal gray area and continually at risk of raids and legal repercussions.

Indeed, the club did face multiple police raids and was eventually shut down in 1998. However, its impact extended far beyond its operational years. It set the stage for Proposition 215, the Compassionate Use Act, which Dennis Peron coauthored. Passed in 1996, this made California the first state to legalize medical cannabis.

The San Francisco Cannabis Buyers Club remains an emblematic institution in the history of medical cannabis in the United States. It showcased the potent combination of community activism, compassion, and "civil disobedience," challenging the norms of its time and paving the way for a broader acceptance of cannabis as medicine.

1996 A Turning Point

In the latter half of the twentieth century, the cannabis narrative began to evolve from stigmatization and demonization to a more distinct and compassionate understanding of its therapeutic potential. The year 1996 stands out as a watershed moment in this shift.

Pioneers like "Brownie Mary" Rathbun and Dennis Peron were instrumental in this transformation. "Brownie Mary" earned her nickname through her compassionate act of distributing homemade cannabis-infused brownies to AIDS patients in San Francisco during the 1980s and 90s. The significant relief these brownies provided to patients, in terms of pain alleviation and appetite stimulation, made their therapeutic value unmistakable.

Dennis Peron, who witnessed firsthand the profound therapeutic effects of cannabis during the AIDS crisis, established the previously mentioned San Francisco Cannabis Buyers Club, the nation's first public marijuana dispensary.

Their collective efforts were pivotal in the passing of Proposition 215 in California, also known as the Compassionate Use Act of 1996. This historic act made California the first US state to legally recognize the medicinal value of cannabis, allowing patients access with a physician's recommendation. Despite this monumental step, the American perception of cannabis was deeply entrenched in decades of stigma, propaganda, and misrepresentation. For many politicians and policy-makers, outdated notions from the era of "Reefer Madness" and the War on Drugs clouded their judgment.

The vilification campaign against cannabis had been so effective that, notwithstanding an increasing body of evidence underscoring its medicinal attributes, a significant portion of the political spectrum remained deeply resistant. However, as more states embarked on their own journeys to acknowledge and adopt medical cannabis programs, it became increasingly challenging to dismiss the growing testimonials of its efficacy. Stories of children experiencing dramatic reductions in epileptic seizures, veterans achieving relief from PTSD, and cancer patients managing their chemotherapy side effects better, began to reshape the narrative.

It's clear that the early efforts of individuals like "Brownie Mary" and Dennis Peron sowed the seeds for a burgeoning movement that questioned long-held misconceptions and championed the medicinal virtues of cannabis.

2000–2018: A Shift in the Cannabis Discourse

As the new millennium dawned, a global reevaluation of cannabis began, driven by a combination of scientific research, patient testimonials, and shifting public opinion. Medical cannabis became the primary catalyst for this change. The plant's therapeutic potential, given the burial of centuries of information, became relegated to anecdotal tales. But with more access to information due to the internet, personal computers, and mobile devices, the narrative of cannabis started to find robust backing in scientific studies, prompting legislative changes in numerous jurisdictions.

In 2001, Canada distinguished itself on the world stage by becoming one of the first nations to nationally legalize medical cannabis. This move not only allowed patients to access cannabis products from licensed producers but also allowed them to grow their own plants in certain cases. The Canadian decision was revolutionary and set a precedent that would resonate across the globe.

Inspiration from such groundbreaking shifts was evident in the US as states like California had pioneered medical cannabis pathways since the late '90s, a cascade of other states, from the Atlantic to the Pacific, began to follow suit. This gradual acceptance of medical cannabis in turn opened the floodgates to discussions around full-blown legalization for adult use.

In the meantime, the US government, specifically the Department of Health and Human Services, was granted a patent for cannabinoids as antioxidants and neuroprotectants in 2003. The patent is numbered 6,630,507. The existence of this patent has been a point of contention for many cannabis advocates, as it appears to acknowledge the medicinal properties of cannabinoids while the federal government simultaneously classified cannabis as a Schedule I substance, suggesting it has "no accepted medical use" (more on this topic in chapter 5).

Uruguay, in 2013, positioned itself at the forefront of this wave, becoming the first country to fully legalize the production, sale, and consumption of cannabis. Their progressive stance was aimed not just at giving citizens freedom of choice but also as a strategic blow to drug cartels, emphasizing regulation over prohibition.

But it was in the US, traditionally the stronghold of the global War on Drugs, that some of the most radical changes were observed. Colorado and Washington, in 2012, set a new course by legalizing recreational cannabis. Their trailblazing move was soon echoed by California, a state with a rich cannabis advocacy history, which voted overwhelmingly in favor of Proposition 64 in 2016.

The implications of these state-level decisions resonated far beyond US borders. By 2018, Canada, building upon its earlier medical cannabis framework, took the audacious step to become the first G7 country to legalize recreational cannabis.

Parallel to these changes, there was growing interest in CBD, a cannabis compound known for its therapeutic benefits without inducing a "high." Recognizing its potential, the 2018 US Farm Bill, signed by President Trump, removed hemp-derived CBD from the list of controlled substances. This was another significant nod to the evolving understanding of cannabis and its constituents.

Across oceans and continents, nations were witnessing these shifts and beginning their own journeys. Whether it was Germany's medical marijuana program, South Africa's move to decriminalize personal use, or Mexico's courts challenging the very legality of cannabis prohibition, the period between 2000 and 2018 marked a turning point. The era will be etched in history as the time the world took a more logical approach to cannabis, recognizing its potential not as a societal menace but as a valuable therapeutic, economic resource, an avenue for the pursuit of social justice reform, and a catalyst for social equity for the communities impacted by the War on Drugs and prohibition.

2020 Cannabis's Elevated Status During a Global Crisis

Amid the global COVID-19 pandemic in 2020, a significant upgrade occurred in the way cannabis was regarded, especially in the United States. As the nation grappled with lockdowns and health concerns, many businesses were forced to close to prevent the spread of the virus. Yet, in several states, cannabis dispensaries were declared "essential businesses," aligning them with other crucial services like grocery stores and pharmacies.

This recognition marked a monumental step in the ongoing journey of cannabis normalization. For a plant that remained "illegal" at the federal level, had been stigmatized, and whose consumers and dealers continued to be incarcerated, the "essential" designation was a testament to how far public perception and policy had evolved, yet it managed to remain an oxymoron. An essential business, with no access to banking...Nonetheless, the "essential designation" acknowledgment underscored the importance of medical cannabis for thousands of patients relying on it for relief from various ailments.

It also emphasized the economic value and job creation associated with the cannabis industry. By 2020, the regulated industry had generated thousands of jobs and contributed significantly to state revenues, making its role even more prominent during a time of economic downturn.

The declaration of cannabis as an essential business during such an unprecedented crisis highlighted the plant's multifaceted significance: medical, economic, and societal. It also provided yet another perspective to consider in the ongoing dialogue surrounding cannabis and its place in modern society.

2024 Closer Than Ever

In a groundbreaking move that promises to transform the American cannabis industry, the U.S. Drug Enforcement Administration (DEA) has shifted its long-standing stance on cannabis. On April 30th, 2024, according to the Associated Press, five anonymous sources with inside knowledge revealed that the DEA's decision aligns with a recommendation from federal health regulators made in August 2023. This pivotal recommendation involves reclassifying cannabis from a Schedule I to a Schedule III substance under the Controlled Substances Act. This reclassification marks a significant recognition of the plant's medical benefits.

On May 16, 2024, US President Joe Biden announced that the Department of Justice (DOJ) would begin the process of reclassifying cannabis to a Schedule III substance within the Controlled Substances Act. This move represents the most significant change in federal drug policy in decades. As the process unfolds, we eagerly await the next steps in this monumental shift.

Where Do We Go from Here?

The landscape of cannabis has evolved significantly over the years, transitioning from a stigmatized and maligned substance to one being widely recognized for its therapeutic potential. The momentum behind cannabis advocacy is undeniable. With each passing year, scientific research underscores its medicinal benefits, eroding long-held prejudices and misconceptions.

Decades ago, the narrative surrounding cannabis was dominated by its prohibition. The journey since then has seen it re-labeled from a forbidden substance to a controlled one. Now, the tides are shifting further, propelled by a growing awareness of its vast potential as medicine, as a viable product, and as a growing industry. Legislation is gradually catching up with the times, reflecting this more enlightened perspective. And with each amendment in policy and each groundbreaking study, the path toward acceptance and normalization of cannabis becomes clearer.

The question isn't if cannabis will be universally accepted but rather when and how. As we move forward, it's essential to continue informed, open dialogues, prioritize scientific exploration, and ensure policies are established with both equity and public health in mind. The future of cannabis is not just about its consumption but about harnessing the plant's full potential for the benefit of all.

Chapter 4
Global Uprooting

The legal status of cannabis has often fluctuated, with many countries having gone through periods of legalization, decriminalization, and re-criminalization. The global trend toward cannabis prohibition was less about the intrinsic properties of cannabis and more about the social, political, and economic contexts of the time. Each country that moved toward prohibition did so for its own specific set of reasons, often influenced by a combination of domestic concerns and international pressures.

The United Nations (UN)

The United Nations (UN) plays a pivotal role in international drug policy, including cannabis reform. The UN's stance on cannabis and other drugs is primarily governed through various international treaties, which member states are encouraged to adopt into their national laws.

Key points regarding the UN and cannabis include:

- *Single Convention on Narcotic Drugs (1961)*: This is one of the most influential international treaties concerning drug control. The convention placed cannabis under Schedule IV, the category for the most dangerous substances. It called for the prohibition of the production and supply of cannabis, except for medical and research purposes.

- *Convention on Psychotropic Substances* (1971): This treaty expanded the international drug control regime to include synthetic and natural psychotropic substances. While its primary focus was on substances like LSD and MDMA, its regulations also impacted the control of cannabis-related substances.
- *United Nations Office on Drugs and Crime* (UNODC): The UNODC is a key UN agency in the fight against illicit drugs, including cannabis. It helps implement the international drug control treaties, offers legal assistance, and works in drug abuse prevention and health.
- *Changes in Global Attitude:* In recent years, there has been a shift in attitudes toward cannabis globally, with an increasing number of countries legalizing or decriminalizing it for medical or recreational use. This shift has put pressure on the UN to reevaluate its stance on cannabis.
- *Reclassification of Cannabis* (2020): In a landmark decision in December 2020, the UN Commission on Narcotic Drugs (CND) voted to remove cannabis from Schedule IV of the 1961 Single Convention on Narcotic Drugs. This was a significant development, acknowledging the medical benefits of cannabis.
- *Impact on Member States:* While UN drug treaties set a framework, they leave room for some flexibility in how countries implement their drug policies. This means that while the UN's stance on cannabis influences global policy, individual countries can and do make their own decisions regarding cannabis legalization or decriminalization.

- *Ongoing Debate:* The debate on the role of cannabis within the UN drug control system continues, reflecting the evolving understanding of the substance's risks and benefits and the changing social and political attitudes toward it worldwide.

The UN's role in cannabis regulation highlights the complexities of international drug policy, balancing between public health, law enforcement, human rights, and scientific research.

Latin America

The global landscape of cannabis legality is a patchwork of different laws, reflecting a range of cultural, social, and political attitudes toward the plant. In Latin America, the history of cannabis legislation varies significantly across countries, with many initially following the lead of the United States in prohibition. Here's an overview of when some key Latin American countries made cannabis illegal:

- *Mexico:* As mentioned earlier, Mexico was one of the first countries to ban cannabis, doing so in 1920. This was part of a larger trend of regulating substances and was influenced by social and political factors.
- *Brazil:* Cannabis was prohibited in Brazil in 1938, under the influence of international drug control treaties and domestic policy.
- *Argentina:* Cannabis was first restricted in Argentina in 1921, with further regulations in the 1930s as part of broader narcotics control efforts.
- *Colombia:* Cannabis became illegal in Colombia in the 1930s, aligning with international narcotics control policies, and legalized for medical use in 2016.
- Chile: In Chile, cannabis was added to the list of controlled substances in 1965.

- *Uruguay:* Interestingly, Uruguay never actually criminalized the possession of drugs for personal use, including cannabis. However, the sale and cultivation were controlled and effectively prohibited until the significant move toward legalization in 2013.
- *Peru:* Cannabis was made illegal in Peru in the 1950s, again influenced by international drug control agreements.
- *Venezuela:* Cannabis prohibition in Venezuela dates back to 1956.
- *Costa Rica:* Cannabis has been illegal in Costa Rica since 1923.
- *Cuba:* Cannabis was banned in Cuba in the 1950s, with strict anti-drug laws following the revolution.
- *In my country, the Dominican Republic,* cannabis was made illegal in 1971 with the enactment of Law 50-88 on Drugs and Controlled Substances. This law was part of a broader trend in the Caribbean and Latin America during the late twentieth century, aligning with global movements toward stricter drug regulations. The law classified marijuana (cannabis) along with other drugs as controlled substances and set penalties for their possession, use, and trafficking.

The Dominican Republic's approach to cannabis and other drugs has historically been influenced by international drug control policies and its relationship with major powers, such as the United States, which has played a significant role in shaping drug policy in the region. Despite this, like many other countries, the Dominican Republic has seen ongoing debates about the potential decriminalization or legalization of cannabis, particularly for medical use. However, as of February 2024, cannabis remains illegal in the Dominican Republic.

These dates and policies reflect the influence of both domestic political and social contexts as well as international drug control treaties and pressures. More recently, there has been a shift in several

Latin American countries toward more liberal policies regarding cannabis, including decriminalization and legalization efforts, as seen in Uruguay and Mexico.

Africa

The illegalization of cannabis in African countries is a complex and diverse subject, reflecting a range of cultural, social, and colonial influences. In many African countries, the initial push toward the illegalization of cannabis was influenced by colonial powers. For example, South Africa, under British rule, was one of the first countries to prohibit cannabis with the 1922 Medical, Dental, and Pharmacy Act. Additionally, post-colonial Africa saw continued influence from international drug control treaties, such as the 1961 Single Convention on Narcotic Drugs, which many African countries ratified, aligning their laws with global narcotics policies.

- *Egypt:* Egypt played a significant role in advocating for the inclusion of cannabis in international drug control conventions in the early twentieth century. Cannabis was restricted in Egypt in the 1920s. Cannabis is illegal in Egypt, and while it is relatively widely used, penalties for possession or trafficking can be harsh.
- *Morocco:* While technically illegal since the early twentieth century, cannabis cultivation has been widespread and partially tolerated, particularly in the Rif region. Morocco is known to be one of the world's largest producers and suppliers of Hashish.
- *Nigeria:* Cannabis was banned in Nigeria in the 1930s, and the country currently has strict laws against its use.
- *Ethiopia:* Despite a long history of traditional use, cannabis is illegal in Ethiopia, although the exact year of its prohibition is not clearly documented.

- *Kenya:* Cannabis was outlawed in Kenya in the 1930s, influenced by both colonial laws and later by international agreements.
- *Ghana:* While traditional use of cannabis has been prevalent, it was made illegal in the 1960s.
- *Lesotho:* In Lesotho, cannabis has been illegal, but it is widely grown and used. Lesotho became the first African country to legalize the cultivation of cannabis for medicinal purposes in 2017.
- *South Africa:* After a long history of prohibition, South Africa made a groundbreaking legal decision in 2018 when the Constitutional Court ruled that the private use and cultivation of cannabis by adults in private spaces is legal.
- *Zimbabwe:* In 2018, Zimbabwe became the second African country to legalize cannabis for medical and scientific purposes.
- *Uganda:* In 1902, the British banned "opium" in Uganda. According to the Eastern Uganda, an Ethnological Survey by Charles William Hobley, as defined by law, opium also included bhang, ganja, churus, and chandoo natron. Uganda legalized cannabis in May 2023 via the Constitutional Court after the law prohibiting its use was nullified.
- *Malawi:* Although illegal, the cannabis plant grows in the wild in many areas of the East African country. Malawian cannabis, particularly the strain known as Malawi Gold, is internationally acclaimed as one of the finest sativa-leaning strains hailing from the African continent. In February 2020, Malawi legalized the cultivation of hemp — the non-psychoactive part of the cannabis plant — as an alternative to tobacco farming.
- *Zambia:* In 2017, Zambia's Minister of Home Affairs clarified that it is legal to cultivate cannabis for medical use with a license from the Department of Health. That same

year, the head of the Department of Health stated that he had no intention of issuing any cultivation licenses.

The situation across the African continent is varied. In some countries, traditional and cultural use of cannabis has conflicted with legal restrictions. In recent years, there has been a shift in some African countries toward exploring the economic and medical potential of cannabis, leading to changes in legislation, particularly regarding medicinal cannabis. However, in many African countries, cannabis remains illegal with strict enforcement of these laws.

Europe

The legal status of cannabis in European countries has evolved over time, with each country having its own unique history and approach to cannabis legislation. Below is an overview of when some key European countries made cannabis illegal and their current stance:

- *United Kingdom:* Cannabis was made illegal in the UK in 1928 as an addition to the Dangerous Drugs Act of 1920. It's currently classified as a Class B drug under the Misuse of Drugs Act 1971. In 2004, the United Kingdom made cannabis a Class C drug with less severe penalties, but it was moved back to Class B in 2009.
- *France:* Cannabis was prohibited in France in 1953. It remains illegal, although there is some movement toward medicinal use.
- *Germany:* Cannabis was first restricted in Germany under the Opium Law of 1929. In April 2024, Germany made it legal for adults to possess 25 grams or less of cannabis in public, up to 50 grams of dried cannabis in private, and grow a maximum of three cannabis plants at home. Adult-only non-profit cannabis social clubs are due to be legalized in Germany in July 2024.

- *Netherlands:* The Netherlands has a unique policy; while cannabis is technically illegal (since 1928), it's decriminalized for personal use, and it's sold in "coffee shops" under certain conditions.
- *Portugal:* Portugal decriminalized the possession of all drugs, including cannabis, for personal use in 2001, although it remains illegal to sell or produce it.
- *Spain:* Spain allows the private consumption and cultivation of cannabis, but public consumption and commercial sales are illegal. Cannabis clubs have a legal gray area where they operate in certain regions.
- *Italy:* Cannabis was banned in Italy in 1923. Medical cannabis is legal and regulated, but recreational use is still illegal, although possession for personal use has been decriminalized.
- *Switzerland:* In Switzerland, cannabis with a THC content of less than 1% is legal. Higher-THC cannabis was made illegal in 1951.
- *Denmark:* Cannabis is illegal in Denmark, though the country has a program for medical cannabis. The Freetown of Christiania in Copenhagen is known for its cannabis trade, but this is technically illegal.
- *Sweden:* Sweden has some of the strictest drug laws in Europe, with cannabis being illegal since 1968.
- *Russia:* Cannabis is illegal in Russia, with laws being particularly strict against drug possession and use.
- *Greece:* Greece made cannabis illegal in 1890. Medical cannabis was legalized in 2017, but recreational use remains illegal.
- *Malta:* In 2018, the Parliament of Malta legalized medical cannabis. On 14 December 2021, the Parliament of Malta legalized recreational cannabis for personal possession and use for those 18-years-old and over, becoming the first EU country to do so.

Each European country has taken a unique path in terms of cannabis legislation. Some countries have decriminalized or legalized medical cannabis, while others maintain strict prohibition. The European landscape continues to evolve with ongoing debates and policy changes regarding cannabis use.

Caribbean

Cannabis legislation in Caribbean countries has historically been influenced by a mix of colonial legacies, international drug treaties, and local cultural practices. Here's an overview of the cannabis situation in some key Caribbean nations:

- *Jamaica:* Jamaica is well-known for its association with cannabis, largely due to Rastafarian culture. Cannabis was illegal in Jamaica for many years (since 1913), but in 2015, the government decriminalized possession of small amounts and legalized it for medical, therapeutic, and religious uses.
- *Trinidad and Tobago:* Cannabis was illegal in Trinidad and Tobago for much of the twentieth century. However, in 2019, the country decriminalized possession of up to 30 grams and allowed the cultivation of up to four plants per household.
- *Barbados:* Barbados legalized medical cannabis in 2019, but recreational use remains illegal. The government is considering further reforms to the cannabis laws.
- *The Bahamas:* In the Bahamas, cannabis remains illegal, and possession can result in severe penalties. There have been discussions about reform, but no significant changes have been made in the last few years.
- *Saint Vincent and the Grenadines:* This country legalized medical cannabis in 2018 and has been exploring the

potential of the cannabis industry for economic development.

- *Dominican Republic:* As previously mentioned, cannabis remains illegal in the Dominican Republic.
- *Cuba:* As previously mentioned, Cuba has strict anti-drug laws, and cannabis remains illegal.
- *Puerto Rico:* As a territory of the United States, Puerto Rico has legalized medical cannabis, but recreational use remains illegal.
- *Antigua and Barbuda:* In 2018, Antigua and Barbuda decriminalized the possession of up to 15 grams of cannabis and allowed households to cultivate up to four plants.
- *Guyana:* Cannabis remains illegal in Guyana, although there has been some discussion about potential decriminalization.

Each Caribbean country's approach to cannabis reflects a balance between cultural attitudes, economic considerations, and international legal obligations. The region has seen a trend toward decriminalization and legalization, especially for medical and religious use, but the legal status and enforcement of cannabis laws can vary significantly from one country to another.

Asia

Many Asian nations have historically had strict anti-cannabis laws with severe penalties, but recent years have seen a shift in some places toward more lenient or reformed policies:

- *China:* As discussed in the first couple of chapters of the book, China has a long history of cannabis cultivation, primarily for industrial hemp, and maintains strict laws against recreational cannabis use. However, it is one of the world's largest producers of hemp.

- *India:* Cannabis has a long cultural history in India, and while recreational use is officially illegal, certain preparations like bhang (a traditional cannabis-infused beverage) are legally and culturally accepted in some parts of the country. Medicinal and industrial hemp use is also being explored more recently.
- *Thailand:* Thailand has taken significant steps in cannabis reform, becoming the first Asian country to legalize medical marijuana in 2018. In 2021, Thailand decriminalized the cultivation and possession of cannabis, though public consumption can still result in penalties, and the sale of cannabis products with high THC content is regulated. After becoming fully legal in 2022, the current Thai government has expressed intentions of going back to a medical-only state.
- *South Korea:* South Korea strictly prohibits recreational cannabis use but broke new ground in East Asia by legalizing medical cannabis in 2018 with tight regulations.
- *Japan:* Japan has stringent anti-cannabis laws with severe penalties for possession, sale, and use. There is little movement toward legalization or decriminalization.
- *Philippines:* The Philippines has harsh drug laws, and cannabis remains illegal. There have been discussions about medical cannabis legalization, but broader drug policy is characterized by a stringent anti-drug stance.
- *Malaysia:* Malaysia has historically had very strict drug laws, including the death penalty for certain drug trafficking offenses. However, there has been some discussion about medical cannabis legalization following high-profile cases.
- *Singapore:* Singapore maintains some of the strictest drug laws in the world, with severe penalties for cannabis possession, use, and trafficking, including the death penalty for high-volume trafficking.

- *Nepal:* Cannabis was traditionally used in Nepal and was legal until the 1970s. While it remains illegal, there have been calls for legalization, and the country has hosted legal cannabis festivals in the past.

The legal landscape for cannabis in the western Pacific is varied and rapidly changing in some regions. While most countries maintain strict controls, the recent shifts, particularly in countries like Thailand and South Korea, indicate a growing openness to medicinal cannabis under regulated conditions.

Middle East

In Middle Eastern countries, the stance on cannabis is generally strict, reflecting conservative societal norms and legal frameworks that often impose severe penalties for possession, use, and trafficking. However, the situation varies by country:

- *Israel:* Israel is a leader in medical cannabis research and has a well-developed medical cannabis program. Recreational use remains illegal, but the country has decriminalized possession of small amounts, shifting toward fines and treatment rather than criminal prosecution.
- *Lebanon:* Lebanon became the first Arab country to legalize cannabis cultivation for medical and industrial use in 2020 in a move to boost its economy. Recreational use remains illegal.
- *Turkey:* Turkey has strict laws against recreational cannabis use but has allowed controlled cultivation of hemp in certain regions for industrial purposes. It has also started to use cannabis-derived medicines under strict regulations.
- *Iran:* Iran has harsh penalties for drug trafficking, including

capital punishment. Cannabis possession and use are illegal, and penalties can be severe.

- *United Arab Emirates (UAE):* The UAE has zero tolerance for drug offenses, including very strict penalties for possession of even trace amounts of cannabis.
- *Saudi Arabia:* Saudi Arabia also enforces strict laws against cannabis, with severe punishments that can include the death penalty for trafficking.
- *Jordan:* Cannabis is illegal in Jordan, and possession or use can result in serious penalties, including imprisonment.
- *Qatar:* Qatar has very strict cannabis laws, with severe penalties for possession, use, or trafficking, including long prison sentences.
- *Oman:* Cannabis is illegal in Oman, with strict laws enforcing penalties for possession, use, and trafficking.

On a personal note, in 2021, I had the pleasure of collaborating with a Lebanese cannabis advocacy group, 420Leb, through a digital event. During this session, I took 420Leb's members on a virtual tour of Jaxx Cannabis Dispensary, showcasing what's possible for Lebanon's commercial cannabis future. We explored the successes and challenges faced in California and the broader US, diving into various business strategies and advocacy efforts. It was enlightening to witness the shared enthusiasm and visions for Lebanon, reaffirming that the cannabis community knows no borders.

In essence, across the Middle East, the approach to cannabis is largely characterized by prohibition and stringent enforcement, though there are exceptions, as seen in Israel's progressive stance on medical cannabis and Lebanon's legalization of cannabis for medical and industrial purposes. It's important to note that there is a global trend toward reevaluating cannabis policies, which could potentially influence changes in this region over time.

Chapter 5
Heroes vs. Villains

As you may have gathered from the last chapter, the origins of the War on Drugs can be traced back to the early twentieth century, when various states and localities in the United States began to pass laws prohibiting the use and sale of drugs such as opium, heroin, cocaine, and cannabis. However, the modern "War on Drugs" is widely considered to have begun in 1971, when President Richard Nixon declared drug abuse to be "public enemy number one" and launched a nationwide campaign "sold" to the American public as a measure to reduce drug use and trafficking in the United States. This initiative involved increased law enforcement efforts, mandatory minimum sentences for drug-related offenses, and the creation of federal drug control agencies such as the DEA. Over the following decades, the War on Drugs continued under subsequent presidents and expanded globally, leading to mass incarceration and controversy over the impact and efficacy of drug criminalization policies.

The War on Drugs has been a continuous battle for the US, consuming trillions of dollars of taxpayer money and militarizing the country's police forces at federal, state, and local levels. Countless lives have been affected in the process, with certain communities, particularly those of Black, Latino, and Native American descent, suffering the absolute most. The campaign has been predominantly conducted in some of the most impoverished and culturally predominantly Black areas of the country, yet the objectives set out by presidents, legislators, law enforcers, and other authorities have been largely unmet, to say the least.

The War on Drugs has been widely considered a failure for several reasons, including:

- *Increased Incarceration Rates*: The War on Drugs has led to a massive increase in the US prison population, with a disproportionate number of nonviolent drug offenders serving extremely long sentences.
- *Racial Disparities*: The War on Drugs has been criticized for disproportionately affecting communities of color, particularly Black Americans, and perpetuating racial inequality in the American criminal justice system and healthcare system.
- *Lack of Effectiveness*: Despite decades of effort and billions of taxpayer dollars spent, the War on Drugs has not reduced drug use or availability.
- *Unintended Consequences*: The War on Drugs has had a number of unintended consequences, such as the reinforcement of black markets and the rise of drug-related violence and criminality.
- *Alternative Approaches*: There is growing evidence that alternative approaches, such as drug education, treatment, and harm reduction initiatives, are more effective and cost-efficient ways of addressing drug-related problems in policing.

Despite its abject failure to protect public health and safety, the War on Drugs has been incredibly successful in one regard: reinforcing systemic racism. The failed war's policies were constructed on race bias and xenophobia. Evidence shows that prohibition enabled the illicit drug trade to flourish, making drugs readily available to adults and adolescents alike while also promoting substance exposure and the likelihood of abuse. In addition, the US criminal justice system has historically discriminated against people of color, imposing an unfair burden on the demographic from the moment of arrest to imprisonment and post-release from prison. This has caused an ongoing cycle of suffering in these respective communities. When will a US president seriously consider updating the way the country handles drug policy and criminalization?

Here's a clear example: the Anti-Drug Abuse Act of 1986 imposed penalties for the possession of crack, a drug often used by disadvantaged and minority communities, that were 100 times harsher than for possession of powder cocaine, a substance more prevalent in wealthier white populations. This act mandated a minimum sentence of five years without parole for possession of 5 grams of crack cocaine, while it mandated the same for possession of 500 grams of powder cocaine. This 100:1 disparity was reduced to 18:1 when crack was increased to 28 grams (1 ounce) by the Fair Sentencing Act of 2010. However, thousands of small-time convicted individuals were excluded from being resentenced due to a "technicality" associated with the Fair Sentencing Act (FSA) of 2010 and its application in subsequent years.

Here is how it went down: first, the Fair Sentencing Act reduced the unfair ratio from 100:1 to 18:1. Then, the First Step Act of 2018 made the Fair Sentencing Act's more lenient penalties retroactive. This meant that individuals who were sentenced before 2010, under the old 100:1 ratio, could potentially have their sentences reduced. Here is the red flag: there was a limitation to this retroactivity. For someone to be eligible for resentencing under the First Step Act, the offender had to have a "covered offense." Congress defined a "covered offense" as "a violation of a federal criminal statute, the statutory penalties for which were modified by section 2 or 3 of the Fair Sentencing Act of 2010... that was committed before August 3, 2010."

In 2021, the US Supreme Court case "Terry v. United States"

examined this issue. The case revolved around Tarahrick Terry, who was arrested in 2008 for possession with intent to distribute 3.9 grams of crack. Terry sought a sentence reduction under the First Step Act, but the lower courts denied it. They found that Terry's crime didn't qualify as a "covered offense" because he was convicted of a low-level crack offense, which wasn't addressed by the Fair Sentencing Act.

The case was taken to the Supreme Court, which upheld the lower court's decision, thereby deciding that the First Step Act's more lenient penalties did not apply to low-level crack offenses. This meant that many individuals, like Terry, convicted of low-level crack offenses before the Fair Sentencing Act's implementation in 2010, could not seek reduced sentences under the First Step Act.

The fight for these disparities continues as in 2021, the US Supreme Court declined to broaden the retroactive resentencing for those affected. The American Civil Liberties Union, the American Conservative Union and related organizations assert that applying the First Step Act retroactively would assist in ending mass incarceration and will reduce its harmful ramifications.

A Tale as Old as Time

Every story has its protagonists and antagonists, and the history of cannabis in the United States is no different. This intricate saga spans decades of fierce advocacy and opposition surrounding the plant's standing within our society.

On the side of progress, advocates championed the myriad benefits of cannabis and hemp. Tirelessly fighting for the rights of patients to access medical cannabis, for the recognition of its wellness properties, for every adult's freedom to choose, and for social justice. These trailblazers' work continues to lay the foundation for the legalization wave we see across many US states and other nations.

In contrast, several political figures and industrialists exploited their influential positions to spearhead campaigns to criminalize cannabis, amplifying racist and damaging narratives about the plant and consumers. These actions not only skewed the criminal justice system, resulting in disproportionate mass incarcerations, particularly affecting Black and Brown communities, but their ripple effects also persist, burdening sectors like the American justice system, healthcare, family welfare, and beyond.

Yet, amid these battles, the resilience of cannabis advocates shines through. Their resolute efforts have made substantial strides in recent years. With an increasing number of states embracing medical and adult-use cannabis programs and decriminalization, it's paramount to honor the legacy of those who championed this cause and those who continue to vouch for its merits.

The following sections within this chapter dive into the prominent figures who have left indelible marks on this ongoing debate, illuminating both the champions and adversaries of the cannabis discourse.

Villains Village

In the complex narrative of cannabis prohibition and its impact on society, several key historical figures emerge who wielded considerable influence in shaping public perception and legislation around cannabis. Among these are Harry J. Anslinger, William R. Hearst, President Nixon, and President Reagan. While their motivations and actions were varied, their collective impact has led to a long-standing and harsh prohibition system that has disproportionately affected and disenfranchised Black and Brown communities. For the context of this section, we have identified some of the "villains" within the cannabis story.

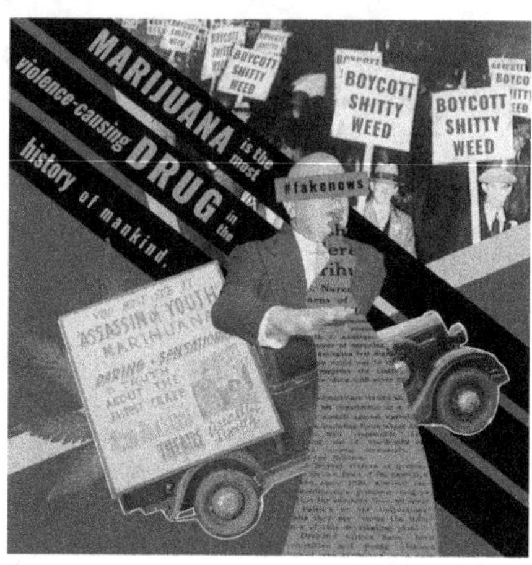

"OG Villain" Graphic by @ProudMaryNetwork for
BSWNation.com

Harry J. Anslinger was a prominent American government official who is known for his role in the criminalization of drug use and the prohibition of cannabis in the United States. He began his career as a government official in 1926 when he was appointed as the Assistant Commissioner of the US Treasury Department's Bureau of Prohibition. In 1930, he was appointed as the first Commissioner of the Federal Bureau of Narcotics (FBN), which was responsible for enforcing federal drug laws.

Anslinger quickly became known for his strong anti-drug stance, particularly when it came to cannabis. He publicized the unfounded message that cannabis was a dangerous substance that posed a threat to public health and safety, and he was determined to see it banned in the United States.

To further this goal, Anslinger used racist and xenophobic rhetoric to associate cannabis use with violence, insanity, and criminal behavior. He propagated the idea that cannabis was a drug used primarily by minorities, particularly African Americans and Mexicans and that its use would lead to societal decay.

Through his position at the FBN, Anslinger successfully lobbied for the passage of the Marihuana Tax Act of 1937, which effectively criminalized cannabis use and possession at the federal level. He continued to push for strict drug laws throughout his career, and his influence on drug policy in the United States has been widely criticized for its racist and discriminatory nature.

We remember Harry J. Anslinger as a controversial figure on the wrong side of history. He played a key role in the criminalization of drug use and the prohibition of cannabis in America. His legacy continues to be felt in drug policy today, and his rhetoric and tactics have been widely criticized for their harmful impact on marginalized communities.

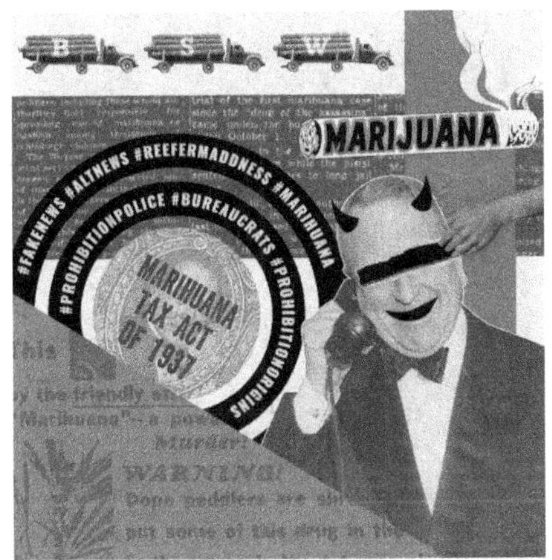

"Fake News King" Graphic by @ProudMaryNetwork for
BSWNation.com

William Randolph Hearst was a wealthy American newspaper publisher born in 1863 in San Francisco, California. He was the owner of several newspapers, including the San Francisco Examiner and the New York Journal.

In the 1930s, the media publications owned by Hearst became known for their racist and inflammatory reporting on cannabis, which was referred to as "marihuana." His newspapers were sources of fear and misinformation about cannabis, particularly among white Americans, who the narrative argued were at risk of being victimized by violent, drug-crazed minorities. Hearst's papers regularly published stories linking cannabis use to violent crime, insanity, and sexual deviance. These media outlets also propagated the idea that cannabis was a drug used primarily by Mexican immigrants and African Americans and that its use would lead to the downfall of American society.

Hearst Media's sensationalistic reporting on cannabis helped to fuel the growing anti-drug hysteria of the 1930s and was instrumental in the passage of the Marihuana Tax Act of 1937, which initiated the snowball effect that evolved into the criminalization cannabis use and possession at the federal level.

Today, Hearst Media's legacy as a newspaper publisher is often overshadowed by his role in the criminalization of cannabis and the perpetuation of harmful racial stereotypes. Their reporting on cannabis is widely criticized for its racist and fear-mongering nature, and his influence on drug policy in the United States has been deeply controversial.

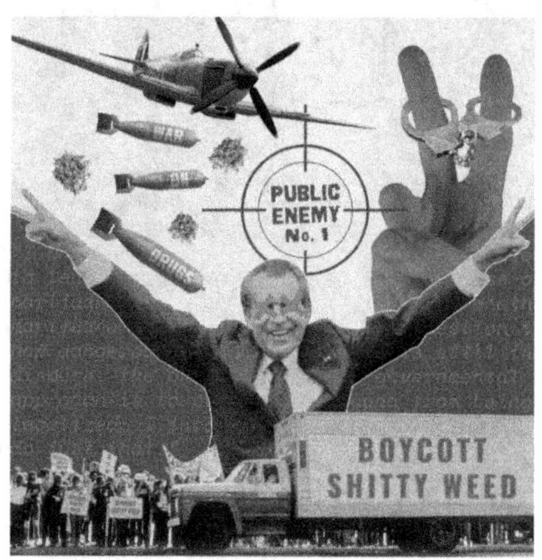

"Public Enemy No. 1" Graphic by @ProudMaryNetwork for BSWNation.com

Richard Nixon was the 37th President of the United States, serving from 1969 to 1974. During his presidency, Nixon launched what would become known as the "War on Drugs" in 1971, which "aimed" to eradicate drug use and drug-related crime in the United States.

Nixon's administration established the DEA in 1973, which was tasked with enforcing federal drug laws and cracking down on drug trafficking. The administration also implemented harsh sentencing guidelines for drug offenses, including mandatory minimum sentences and the use of the death penalty for drug-related crimes.

One of the key targets of Nixon's drug policies was cannabis, which he declared to be a dangerous, highly addictive drug with no medical value. Under his leadership, the Controlled Substances Act of 1970 was passed, which classified cannabis as a Schedule I drug alongside heroin and LSD, effectively criminalizing its use and possession at the federal level.

Nixon's "War on Drugs" was heavily criticized for its disproportionate impact on communities of color and for perpetuating stereotypes about drug use. The policies implemented during his presidency have been widely credited with contributing to the rise of mass incarceration in the United States and have been blamed for exacerbating the opioid epidemic.

Despite this, Nixon's legacy as a staunch advocate of the criminalization of drug use remains influential to this day. Many of the drug policies and laws that were established during his presidency are still in place, and the debate over drug abuse being a healthcare versus a criminal issue continues to be a highly contested issue in American politics.

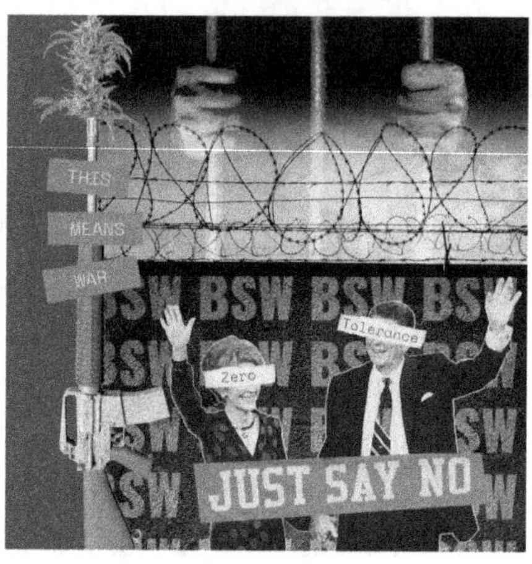

"Zero Tolerance" Graphic by @ProudMaryNetwork for BSWNation.com

Ronald and Nancy Reagan were the 40th President and First Lady of the United States, respectively, serving from 1981 to 1989. During their time in the White House, the Reagans became known for their strong stance against drug use and their efforts to combat it in America.

One of the most famous initiatives that the Reagans launched was the "Just Say No" campaign, which encouraged children and teenagers to resist peer pressure and say no to drugs. This campaign became a cultural phenomenon in the 1980s and was widely adopted by schools and community organizations across the country. In addition to the "Just Say No" campaign, the Reagan administration also implemented a number of policies aimed at cracking down on drug use and drug-related crime. The most notable of these policies was the Anti-Drug Abuse Act of 1986, which established mandatory minimum sentences for drug offenses and created the Office of National Drug Control Policy (ONDCP).

Another key initiative that the Reagans championed was the D.A.R.E. (Drug Abuse Resistance Education) program, which aimed to prevent drug use among young people by educating them about the dangers of drugs and helping them develop resistance to peer pressure. While the program was initially hailed as a success, subsequent studies have shown that it had little to no impact on drug use among young people.

Despite their efforts, the Reagans' approach to drug policy has been widely criticized for its emphasis on criminalization and punishment rather than treatment and prevention. Critics argue that the policies implemented during their presidency disproportionately impacted communities of color and contributed to the rise of mass incarceration in the United States in a major way.

Heroes Haven

Throughout the turbulent history of cannabis, not all characters chose the path of opposition and stigma. Many brave individuals took a stand against the prevailing winds of the time, championing the virtues of the plant and challenging its demonization. Dennis Peron, Bob Marley, Mary Jane Rathbun, Mila Jenkins, and Jack Herer are among those indomitable humans who fervently advocated for cannabis rights. They confronted enormous societal and legal pressures, yet their determination never wavered. They believed in the therapeutic and holistic benefits of cannabis, and in many ways, their relentless advocacy sowed the seeds for the reformation movements we see today. In this section, we delve deep into the lives and legacies of these trailblazers, exploring their challenges, triumphs, and the indelible marks they left on the canvas of cannabis history. These are their stories:

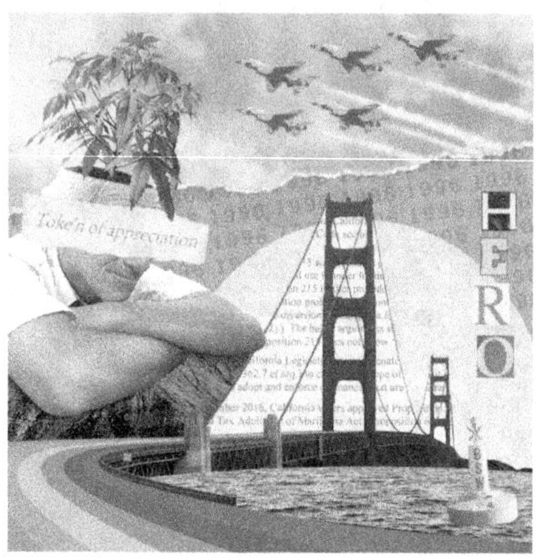

"The Godfather" Graphic by @ProudMaryNetwork for BSWNation.com

Dennis Peron was a prominent American cannabis activist and advocate for the legalization of medical cannabis. He is widely regarded as the "father of cannabis" in California for his tireless efforts in advancing the cause of medical cannabis.

Born on April 8, 1945, in the Bronx, New York, Peron moved to San Francisco in the 1970s, where he became involved in the cannabis movement. He was a founding member of the San Francisco Cannabis Buyers Club, which was the first public medical marijuana dispensary in the United States. In the 1980s and 1990s, Peron played a significant role in advocating for the use of medical cannabis in the LGBTQ+ community at the height of the AIDS epidemic. He witnessed first-hand the benefits of marijuana on patients suffering from AIDS-related illnesses, and he fought tirelessly for the legalization of medical cannabis to help those in need.

In 1996, Peron was one of the main architects of California's Proposition 215, which legalized medical cannabis in the state. He was instrumental in raising awareness about the medical benefits of cannabis and the need for patients to have access to the plant. As discussed in the previous chapter, the SF Cannabis Buyers Club was established to provide medical cannabis to patients with serious illnesses, such as AIDS, cancer, multiple sclerosis, and other conditions. The club operated in a gray area with respect to legalities, as medical cannabis was not yet legal in California or anywhere else in the US at the time. However, Dennis Peron and the members of the Buyer's Club argued that providing medical cannabis to those who needed it was a matter of compassion and public health.

The San Francisco Cannabis Buyers' Club became a rallying point for medical cannabis advocates, who argued that patients should have access to the plant under certain circumstances. The club also provided a model for other medical cannabis dispensaries that opened in California and other states in the following years. The San Francisco Cannabis Buyers' Club is remembered as an important landmark in cannabis advocacy and pioneering in the fight for cannabis legalization.

Throughout his life, Peron remained an outspoken advocate for the legalization of cannabis and continued to work toward this goal until his death in 2018. His legacy continues to inspire those who fight for the rights of medical cannabis patients and for the legalization of marijuana worldwide.

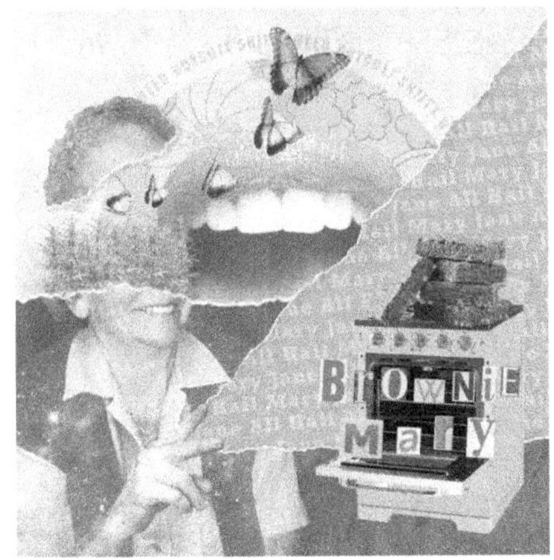

"All Hail Mary Jane" Graphic by @ProudMaryNetwork for
BSWNation.com

Mary Jane Rathbun, also known as Brownie Mary, was a prominent

American cannabis activist and advocate for medical cannabis. She was born in Chicago in 1922 and grew up in Minneapolis before moving to San Francisco in the 1950s.

In the 1980s, Mary became a hospital volunteer at San Francisco General Hospital, where she began baking and distributing cannabis-infused brownies to AIDS patients. She was a compassionate caregiver and believed that medical cannabis could provide relief to those suffering from chronic illnesses. Mary quickly gained a reputation as "Brownie Mary" and became a beloved figure in the medical cannabis community. She was arrested several times for her cannabis activism but remained steadfast in her beliefs and continued to advocate for the legalization of the plant.

In 1991, Mary was awarded the Humanitarian of the Year Award by the San Francisco Board of Supervisors for her work with AIDS patients. She used the award ceremony as a platform to speak out about the need for medical cannabis and urged lawmakers to change their stance on the plant. Mary passed away in 1999 at the age of 77, but her legacy lives on as an inspiration to those fighting for medical cannabis rights. She is remembered as a passionate advocate for compassion and justice who believed in the healing power of cannabis and fought tirelessly for its legalization.

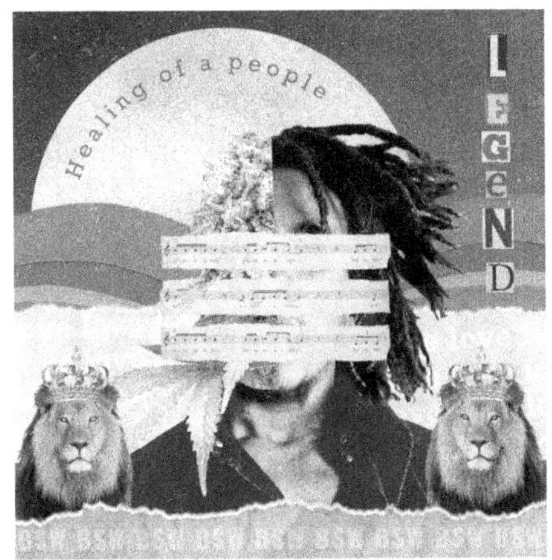

*"Legendary OG" Graphic by @ProudMaryNetwork for
BSWNation.com*

Bob Marley was a Jamaican singer-songwriter and musician who is widely regarded as one of the most iconic and influential musicians of the twentieth century. He was born on February 6, 1945, in St. Ann Parish, Jamaica. In addition to his music career, Bob Marley was also a well-known advocate for cannabis and its use in Rastafarian culture. Rastafarianism is a religion that originated in Jamaica in the 1930s, which holds cannabis as a sacrament and a tool for spiritual enlightenment.

Bob Marley himself was a devout Rastafarian and believed that cannabis played an important role in his spiritual journey. He often spoke publicly about his belief in the benefits of cannabis and its use in Rastafarian culture. Bob Marley's music also reflected his views on cannabis and its role in Rastafarianism. Many of his songs, such as "Kaya" and "Easy Skanking," referenced cannabis and its use in Jamaican culture. Despite facing criticism and persecution for his advocacy of cannabis, Bob Marley remained steadfast in his beliefs and continued to promote the use of cannabis as a tool for spiritual enlightenment and cultural identity.

Today, Bob Marley's legacy as a cannabis advocate and cultural icon continues to inspire those who believe in the healing power of cannabis and the importance of spiritual enlightenment. His music and message of peace, love, and unity continue to resonate with people around the world, making him a true icon of cannabis activism.

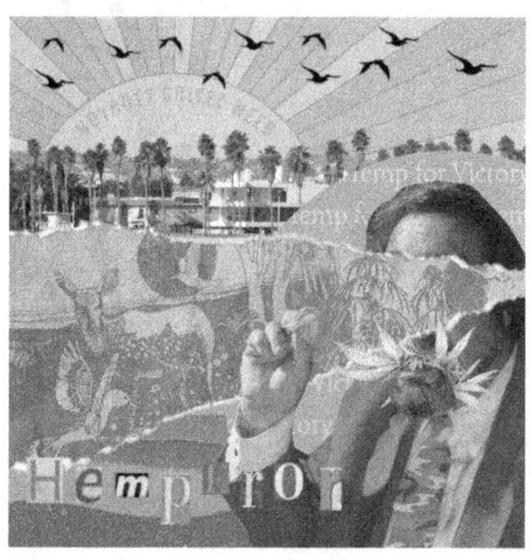

"The Hemperor" Graphic by @ProudMaryNetwork for BSWNation.com

Jack Herer was a prominent American cannabis activist, author, and entrepreneur who is widely regarded as one of the most influential figures in the modern cannabis legalization movement. He was born on June 18, 1939, in New York City.

In 1985, Jack Herer published his book *The Emperor Wears No Clothes*, which is considered a seminal work in the cannabis legalization movement. The book provided a detailed history of the prohibition of cannabis and argued that the plant should be legalized for its many benefits, including its potential as a sustainable and environmentally friendly source of fiber and fuel.

To write the book, Jack Herer conducted extensive research at the Library of Congress, reviewing decades of government-backed research on hemp fiber and cannabis. He became a tireless activist for the legalization of cannabis, traveling the country to speak at rallies and events and lobbying lawmakers to change their stance on the drug.

Jack Herer also founded the Emperor Wears No Clothes Foundation, which promoted hemp and cannabis education and research. He was a vocal advocate for the medical benefits of cannabis and believed that the plant should be legal for both medicinal and recreational use.

In addition to his activism, Jack Herer was also an entrepreneur who started several successful hemp-based businesses, including the first hemp store in the United States. He passed away on April 15, 2010, but his legacy as a cannabis activist and entrepreneur lives on.

Today, Jack Herer is remembered as a passionate advocate for the legalization of cannabis and a visionary who saw the potential of the plant to transform many industries, from textiles to energy. His book, *The Emperor Wears No Clothes*, remains an important work in the cannabis legalization movement and a testament to his dedication and hard work.

Mila Jansen is a legendary figure in the cannabis industry. Known as the "Hash Queen," her life story is nothing short of extraordinary. A free-spirited woman who traversed an unconventional path to become one of the most respected figures in cannabis, Mila's journey is a testament to ingenuity, resilience, and unwavering belief in the power of cannabis.

Born in 1944 in Liverpool, England, Mila moved to Amsterdam at a young age. As a single mother of four in the 1960s, she lived a bohemian lifestyle, opening Amsterdam's first tea house, "The Mellow Yellow," where individuals could openly enjoy cannabis. The tea house soon transformed into one of the first "coffee shops" in Amsterdam, setting the groundwork for the city's now-famous coffee shop culture.

Mila's life took a significant turn during a trip to India in the 1970s, where she was introduced to the practice of making hand-rubbed hashish. Intrigued by the process and the potential of creating high-quality hashish, she embarked on a quest to perfect the craft. This interest led to her revolutionary invention: a simple, effective hash-making device that came to be known as "The Pollinator."

The Pollinator was a game-changer in cannabis extraction, allowing for efficient, high-yield production of hashish. It utilized a rotating drum and a sieve to separate the trichomes from the plant material, the first of its kind to do so. The invention was an instant success and paved the way for her future developments, including the Ice-O-Lator and the Bubbleator, which further revolutionized the hash-making process.

Despite facing numerous hurdles, including legal issues and societal stigma, Mila continued her pioneering work in cannabis. Her contributions have significantly shaped modern cannabis extraction techniques, and she has played a key role in advancing the acceptance and understanding of cannabis, particularly in terms of its medicinal properties.

Mila's dedication to the craft of hashish making and her advocacy for the cannabis plant have not only earned her the title of "Hash Queen" but also the respect and admiration of the cannabis community worldwide. Now in her seventies, Mila continues to be an influential figure, sharing her wealth of knowledge through workshops, speaking engagements, and her autobiography, "How I Became the Hash Queen."

Mila's story serves as an inspiration for many in the cannabis industry, a testament to the power of innovation and the spirit of resilience. Despite the challenges, she remained undeterred, driven by her belief in the therapeutic potential of cannabis and her desire to make high-quality hashish accessible to all. Her pioneering efforts have undoubtedly left an indelible mark on the industry, shaping the way cannabis is processed and consumed today.

Elvy Musikka. In the complex saga of cannabis activism, personal stories often resonate louder than statistics or policies. Elvy Musikka's tale is a prime example. In 1976, the same year Robert Randall celebrated a landmark medical necessity victory in Judge Washington's court, Elvy chanced upon the benefits of marijuana for her eyes. Empowered by Robert's triumph and driven by personal necessity, she researched fervently, even following her doctor's recommendation to try marijuana-infused brownies. To her delight, they worked. For over a decade, her condition remained stable, prompting her to cultivate her own marijuana plants, ensuring an uninterrupted supply.

However, 1988 brought a dramatic twist. Elvy's cultivation led to her arrest. Without hesitation, she reached out to Robert, a connection she had anticipated for years. Preparing for her court battle, Elvy faced many challenges. Her primary ophthalmologist was initially hesitant but eventually chose to stand beside her in court. With Robert's guidance and assistance from NORML's attorney, Norm Kent, they crafted a robust defense based on medical necessity.

In a courtroom in Broward County, Florida, a significant moment unfolded. After a non-jury trial, Judge Mark E. Polen, in a notable verdict, sided with Musikka. His declaration: "I don't see where a better case could ever be made for medical necessity. Miss Musikka is trying to preserve herself from serious bodily injury."

Elvy's victory didn't end there. She applied and was granted access to the federal Compassionate IND program, making her the second woman, after Anne Guttentag in 1980, to receive federal marijuana supplies. However, while Guttentag tragically received her supply too late for effective treatment, Elvy's journey bore more fruit. For over two decades, this federal supply played a pivotal role in preserving her vision. Beyond personal benefits, Elvy used her position to champion the cause, eventually opting for legal cannabis from her new home in Oregon over the federal supply.

Elvy's case marked a significant milestone, being the first successful medical necessity plea in Florida and only the third in the nation. While using the medical necessity defense was intricate and required a precise alignment of conditions, those like Elvy who succeeded with this plea etched essential chapters in the broader tale of medical cannabis reform.

Todd McCormick emerges as a bona fide survivor during the pivotal years following California's Proposition 215 raids by the federal government despite the state's legalization of medical cannabis. Enacted in 1996, this groundbreaking legislation gave the green light to medical marijuana in the Golden State. McCormick wasn't just an armchair advocate; he was on the front lines, championing cannabis as a lifeline for people dealing with cancer, AIDS, and chronic pain.

But in 1997, McCormick's actions landed him in hot water. Even though Prop 215 was California law, federal statutes still criminalized cannabis cultivation. McCormick, caught growing an eye-popping 4,000 cannabis plants, found himself facing federal charges. Trapped in the clutches of a federal courtroom, he was prohibited by the judge to invoke Prop 215 as a defense.

McCormick's arrest and subsequent five-year sentence in federal prison served as a wake-up call, underscoring the jarring disconnect between state and federal cannabis laws, a hot mess we're still untangling today. But rather than disappearing into the archives of cannabis history, McCormick became a touchstone in the fight for reform. He leveraged his story to spark conversations, rally activists, and educate the public about cannabis's medicinal value and the glaring need for more research.

McCormick is still out there, banging the drum for the recognition of cannabis as medicine and as a valuable crop. His life serves as a compelling case study of the complexities and absurdities of America's drug policy—a testament to the rocky road toward cannabis re-legalization and acceptance. Put simply, McCormick embodies the heroism threaded throughout the evolving narrative of cannabis in the United States.

Keith Stroup. In the complicated tapestry of cannabis activism and policy reform, few names shine as brightly as Keith Stroup, the founder of NORML. If Todd McCormick is a frontline soldier in the battle for cannabis legalization, Stroup is a strategist, one of the individuals who took up the banner of reform not just for a season but for a lifetime. His story, rich in both triumphs and setbacks, is a mirror reflecting the broader struggle for cannabis reform in the United States.

In 1970, a young Stroup founded NORML with a clear but audacious mission: to move public opinion sufficiently to achieve the decriminalization of cannabis for adult use. Back in the early '70s, this idea seemed almost laughably utopian. Cannabis was a Schedule I drug, sharing the category with substances like heroin. The public sentiment was influenced by a barrage of anti-drug campaigns, and the judicial system was suffocating under the weight of draconian drug laws. It was a bleak landscape for any reform, let alone cannabis. But Stroup was undeterred.

Harnessing the momentum of the anti-Vietnam protests and the civil rights movement, Stroup managed to tap into a burgeoning countercultural spirit that questioned authority and demanded change. NORML began its journey as a scrappy but vocal advocate, taking up litigation cases that challenged cannabis arrests, launching public awareness campaigns, and lobbying tirelessly at the state and federal levels.

It's crucial to remember that NORML was founded the same year that the Controlled Substances Act came into effect, an act that would provide the legislative framework for the War on Drugs. This timing was not coincidental but deeply ironic. While NORML was articulating a vision of reform, the government was doubling down on punitive measures. In that environment, Stroup's organization had to be more than just vocal; it had to be strategic and relentless.

NORML's impact on the discourse around cannabis has been transformative, to say the least. And while the 1980s brought a resurgence of conservative anti-drug policies—Reagan's "Just Say No" campaign comes to mind—NORML persisted, becoming a repository of information, advocacy, and legal support for those entangled in the War on Drugs. More about NORML as an organization in a later chapter.

Keith Stroup wasn't just the organization's founder; he was its heart and soul. Stroup made it his life's work to attend nearly every cannabis event, debate, and legislative session he could. His advocacy work was backed by a keen legal mind—Stroup's background is law. Although he stepped down as NORML's executive director, he continued to serve as legal counsel and remained a prominent voice on the advisory board.

Stroup's influence is particularly remarkable when we consider the social changes he has witnessed and impacted. He saw cannabis go from being a taboo subject to a topic of serious legislative discussion. Today, given how far we have come since 1974, we can feel comfortable saying that Stroup's early vision seems less like a pipe dream and more like a prophecy coming to fruition. Stroup contributions are not just historical footnotes; they are active, living legacies that continue to inform and drive the march toward cannabis re-legalization and normalization. In every sense of the word, Stroup is a pioneer whose efforts will be remembered and celebrated for generations to come.

In the unfolding drama of cannabis in America, heroes come in many forms: patients fighting for medical access, entrepreneurs navigating a labyrinthine regulatory landscape, activists taking to the streets (or the internet), and visionaries plotting a course toward a more equitable and sensible future. There are so many more advocates and organizations who have contributed to the progress that has been made within this movement. There are not enough pages in this book to highlight them all. But we can all start these conversations and give advocates their flowers while they can still smell them. The advocacy work in this space is never over. There is still a lot of work to do and a lot of opportunities to contribute.

Look in the mirror. You are the HERO!

...Then check this out:

BSW NATION METAVERSE
IN SPATIAL.IO

The second collection of my lifestyle brand, Boycott Shitty Weed (www.BSWNation.com), is called propaganda. The collection aims to bring awareness to the origins of prohibition by exposing the historical characters who ignorantly criminalized the cannabis plant and highlights the heroes who devoted their lives to cannabis advocacy work, inciting the origins of legalization in the US. Check out the BSW Nation metaverse on Spatial.io for an immersive experience of this chapter.

Chapter 6
Prohibition Profiteers

Unpacking the Beneficiaries of the Chaos

When society nurtures a population that has access to natural mental and physical health therapies, the results are transformative. People tend to be more creative, less burdened by pain or stress, and less susceptible to addictive behaviors. They sleep better, have elevated spirits, and possess a clearer focus on positivity rather than being consumed by fear or distractions. Such an empowered population, which in my opinion cannabis has the potential to foster, is not easily swayed or dominated.

Yet, certain entrenched interests thrive when the populace remains in the opposite state: docile, distracted, fearful, and in need. These forces capitalize on the very human conditions that holistic therapies like cannabis can address. Key players among these beneficiaries are:

- *Big Pharma*: Dominates the medical landscape, often profiting from prolonged treatments and recurring prescriptions.

- *Big Alcohol:* Fears competition from cannabis, a natural relaxant and mood enhancer.
- Big Tobacco: Despite recent overtures toward the cannabis industry, they have historically seen it as a threat to cigarette sales and, most recently, vape sales.
- *Big Agriculture:* A massive industry that could be disrupted by the widespread cultivation and diverse applications of hemp.
- *Government:* Gains revenue from fines, forfeitures, and other penalties related to drug offenses and propaganda campaigns.
- *Correctional Facilities System:* Profits from the high rates of incarceration are linked to drug offenses big and small, especially those tied to cannabis.

The mosaic of cannabis prohibition is multifaceted, with various stakeholders benefiting from the status quo. The web of interests that sustains cannabis's criminalization runs deep. Understanding it is crucial for anyone hoping to untangle and change the present system.

Big Pharma

The Big Pharma industry in the US refers to the largest multinational corporations that produce and sell pharmaceutical drugs. These companies are some of the largest and most profitable corporations in the world, with a significant global market share.

According to Statista, the largest pharmaceutical company in the US by revenue in 2021 was Pfizer Inc., followed by Merck & Co. Inc. and Johnson & Johnson. These companies not only dominate the pharmaceutical industry but also have significant influence in politics and public health policies related to drug development, approval, and pricing.

The pharmaceutical industry is responsible for developing and manufacturing drugs that treat and prevent diseases and illnesses, including both prescription and over-the-counter drugs. According to the Pharmaceutical Research and Manufacturers of America, the industry invested $83 billion in research and development in 2019 alone.

In terms of their economic impact, the pharmaceutical industry generates hundreds of billions of dollars in revenue each year. According to a report by IQVIA, global spending on prescription drugs is expected to reach $1.5 trillion by 2023.

However, the industry has also faced criticism for its high drug prices, its role in the opioid epidemic, and its influence on medical research and healthcare policy. Critics argue that the industry prioritizes profits over public health and that the cost of many drugs is unaffordable for many patients.

Cannabis legalization is a threat to Big Pharma. The pharmaceutical industry is one of the biggest beneficiaries of cannabis prohibition, as they currently can market and sell their own drugs legally, no matter the side effects. From the outside looking in, to Big Pharma, it is all about the money.

Ok, but how does Big Pharma benefit from cannabis prohibition?

Well, first, prohibition prevents the legal and widespread use of cannabis as a medicine, which allows pharmaceutical companies to market and sell their own alternative drugs; for example, the FDA-approved cannabis-derived drug product Epidiolex (cannabidiol), as well as three synthetic cannabis-related drug products: Marinol (dronabinol), Syndros (dronabinol), and Cesamet (nabilone). These approved drug products are only available with a prescription from a licensed healthcare provider. This creates a captive market for their products and ensures that they remain the dominant players in the healthcare industry when it comes to [synthetic] cannabinoids.

Second, pharmaceutical companies have a financial interest in maintaining the status quo, as cannabis-based medicines could potentially cut into their profits. If cannabis were to become widely available and legal, it could provide patients with an alternative to expensive pharmaceutical drugs, particularly for conditions like chronic pain, anxiety, and sleep disorders. ...Imagine people grew their own medicine?

Third, pharmaceutical companies also benefit from the current regulatory environment, which places strict controls on the development and testing of cannabis-based medicines. The regulatory barriers to entry in this field are high, which limits competition and ensures that pharmaceutical companies remain the primary suppliers of (synthetic) cannabis-based drugs.

The pharmaceutical industry benefits from cannabis prohibition by maintaining its dominant position in the healthcare industry, ensuring a captive market for its products, and limiting competition from alternative treatments.

#RedFlag

It's important to note that given the strides in legalization, there is now a growing interest in the development of cannabis-based medicines, particularly for the treatment of certain medical conditions by pharmaceutical companies. Big Pharma has access to the capital that the current cannabis industry does not have access to due to the federal status, among other challenges.

Big Alcohol

The big alcohol industry in the US refers to the largest multinational corporations that produce and sell alcoholic beverages. These companies are some of the largest and most profitable corporations in the world, with a significant global market share.

According to Statista, the leading alcohol producer in the United States in 2021 was Anheuser-Busch InBev, with a market share of approximately 45 percent. Other major players in the industry include Molson Coors, Constellation Brands, and Diageo.

These companies not only dominate the alcohol industry but also have a significant influence on politics and public health policies related to alcohol use. They have also been subject to numerous lawsuits and legal challenges related to their marketing practices, as well as the health effects of alcohol consumption.

In terms of their economic impact, the alcohol industry generates billions of dollars in revenue each year. According to the National Institute on Alcohol Abuse and Alcoholism, the total economic cost of alcohol-related problems in the US was estimated to be $249 billion in 2010. This includes costs related to healthcare, lost productivity, and criminal justice.

However, the industry has also faced criticism for its negative impact on public health, including its contribution to the global epidemic of alcohol-related diseases such as liver disease and certain types of cancer, as well as its role in promoting excessive alcohol consumption and alcoholism.

Big alcohol companies benefit from cannabis prohibition in several ways. Prohibition prevents the legal and widespread use of cannabis as a recreational substance, which ensures that alcohol remains the dominant legal intoxicant in society. This creates a captive market for alcohol products and ensures that these companies continue to make profits.

There is money in alcohol, too, as alcohol can be addictive. Cannabis use can potentially cut into the profits of big alcohol companies, particularly in the context of social gatherings and consumption events. If cannabis were to become widely available and legal, it could provide consumers with an alternative to alcohol, particularly for those who are looking to avoid the negative health effects and potential addiction issues associated with alcohol use. Needless to say, cannabis can also be consumed as an infused beverage.

Third, big alcohol companies have a financial interest in maintaining the current regulatory environment, which places strict controls on the sale and distribution of cannabis. This ensures that cannabis remains a controlled substance and limits the possibilities for competition from a potentially disruptive new industry.

#RedFlag

Not all alcohol companies oppose the legalization of cannabis. As a matter of fact, some have a vested interest in public cannabis corporations, and some may even be exploring the development of cannabis-infused products.

Big Tobacco

The big tobacco industry refers to the largest multinational corporations that produce and sell tobacco products. These companies are some of the largest and most profitable corporations in the world, with a significant global market share.

According to Forbes, the biggest tobacco company in the world in 2021 was Philip Morris International, with a market capitalization of over $160 billion. Other major players in the industry include British American Tobacco, Japan Tobacco International, and Altria Group, Inc.

These companies not only dominate the tobacco industry but also have significant influence in politics and public health policies related to tobacco use. They have also been subject to numerous lawsuits and legal challenges related to their marketing practices, as well as the health effects of tobacco use.

In terms of their economic impact, the tobacco industry generates billions of dollars in revenue each year. However, the industry has also faced criticism for its negative impact on public health, including its contribution to the global epidemic of smoking-related diseases such as lung and throat cancer, and heart disease.

Tobacco companies also benefit from the prohibition of cannabis, as it prevents competition from a new industry. If cannabis were to become legal and widely available, it could potentially cut into the profits of these established industries, which have a lot of political power and influence.

- *Maintaining their market share*: By keeping cannabis illegal, big tobacco companies can prevent a potential competitor from entering the market and taking away their market share.
- *Preventing the diversion of users*: Cannabis is often seen as a less harmful alternative to tobacco, and by keeping it illegal, tobacco companies can prevent some of their customers from switching to cannabis products.
- *Maintaining their political power*: Given their access to capital, "big tobacco" companies have significant political influence, and by supporting cannabis prohibition, they can help maintain their political power and prevent potential regulatory challenges to their business.
- *Expanding their product lines*: If cannabis were to become legal, big tobacco companies could potentially enter the market and use their existing infrastructure to produce and distribute cannabis products. However, by keeping cannabis illegal, they can avoid the costs of entering a new market while still benefiting from their existing tobacco products.

#RedFlag

It is worth noting that some big tobacco companies, such as Altria, have already invested in the cannabis industry, recognizing the potential profits that could be made if cannabis becomes legal at the federal level.

Big Agriculture

Other industries, such as big agriculture, may also benefit from cannabis prohibition. For example, hemp, which is a variety of the cannabis plant, has numerous industrial uses and could potentially compete with other agricultural crops. As discussed in an earlier chapter, hemp is a variety of the cannabis plant that has numerous industrial uses, including fiber, paper, textiles, biodegradable plastics, fuel, and construction materials. Hemp can potentially compete with other agricultural crops due to its versatility and potential profitability, particularly in areas where other crops may not grow as well.

While hemp has the potential to compete with other agricultural crops, its regulatory restrictions and requirements can create challenges for farmers and businesses looking to enter the industry. However, as more states and countries regulate hemp production, it is likely that the industry will become more accessible and profitable for those who choose to participate.

Big agriculture, or the large-scale farming operations that dominate the agricultural industry, can benefit from cannabis prohibition in several ways:

- *Monopoly on Textile and Paper Production*: Cannabis, specifically hemp, can be used to produce textiles, paper, and a variety of other products. With cannabis prohibition in place, hemp production is limited or outright banned in many regions, allowing traditional agricultural industries, such as the cotton and timber sectors, to maintain their dominance in textile and paper markets.

- *Reduced Competition*: Hemp is a resilient crop that can grow in various climates with minimal inputs. If widely cultivated, it could potentially offer a more sustainable and cheaper alternative to some traditional crops. By keeping cannabis and hemp illegal or heavily regulated, larger agricultural entities can keep a potentially competitive crop at bay.

- *Control Over New Markets*: If and when cannabis becomes legal, big agriculture, with its vast resources, stands poised to dominate the market quickly. By slowing down or controlling the legalization process, they can strategize their entry and establish a strong foothold once legalization occurs.

- *Pesticide and Herbicide Sales:* Cannabis crops, when grown extensively, may not require the same volume of pesticides and herbicides as some other staple crops, given their natural resistances. This could mean reduced sales for agribusiness companies that produce these chemicals.
- *Leverage Over Research:* Cannabis prohibition has limited the amount of research completed on the plant. Big agriculture, with its extensive resources, has the potential to control or heavily influence the direction of research once the prohibition is lifted, ensuring it aligns with their business interests.
- *Influence Over Legislation:* With the prohibition in place, big agriculture can use its lobbying power to shape any future cannabis-related legislation. This can ensure that any legal framework developed will be to their benefit, potentially by introducing barriers to entry for smaller growers or by securing favorable taxation and subsidy structures.
- *Supply Chain Control:* Prohibition allows big agriculture to invest in and establish robust supply chains for alternative products, ensuring their dominance in the market. Once cannabis is legalized, they could potentially repurpose or expand these supply chains to control cannabis distribution.

Additionally, some large agricultural companies, including those that produce genetically modified crops and agricultural chemicals, may benefit from expensive regulatory requirements for legal cannabis cultivation and production. Expensive regulatory requirements can create a barrier to entry for small-scale growers and cultivators who may not have the financial resources to comply with the regulations. This can limit competition, allowing larger agricultural companies to dominate the market and potentially cause legacy operators to be excluded from the regulated industry. Large agricultural companies may also have the resources to invest in research and development to create new strains of cannabis that meet regulatory requirements and are more resistant to pests and diseases, further consolidating their market power.

The Government

Third, the DEA, FBI, and local law enforcement agencies also benefit from the War on Drugs, as it provides them with a justification for their budgets and resources. These agencies have a vested interest in maintaining the current system, as it allows them to continue to receive funding for drug enforcement efforts.

The DEA, FBI (Federal Bureau of Investigation), and local law enforcement agencies can benefit from the War on Drugs in several ways:

- *Funding:* The War on Drugs has resulted in increased funding for law enforcement agencies, particularly those involved in drug enforcement efforts. This funding can be used to purchase equipment, hire additional staff, and cover other expenses related to drug enforcement initiatives.
- *Asset forfeiture:* Law enforcement agencies can seize assets, such as cash and property, from individuals and organizations involved in drug-related activities. These assets can be used to fund law enforcement operations or sold at auction to generate revenue.
- *Career advancement:* Successful drug enforcement operations can lead to promotions and career advancement for law enforcement personnel, including increased pay and benefits.

- *Political influence:* Law enforcement agencies involved in the War on Drugs can wield significant political influence, particularly in advocating for increased funding and support for drug enforcement efforts.

As we all already know, the War on Drugs has also been criticized for its negative impacts on communities, including disproportionate targeting and incarceration of marginalized groups and the perpetuation of systemic racism. Adding fuel to this fire is the fact that there is an ongoing debate over whether the benefits of the War on Drugs outweigh its costs and negative consequences, yet not much action is taken to make an impactful change for the better.

The US Government's Contradictory Stance: Patenting Cannabinoids

Amid the sweeping prohibition of cannabis, one would expect the US government to distance itself entirely from any association with the plant or its derivatives. Yet, in a twist of irony, the Department of Health and Human Services was granted a patent for cannabinoids as antioxidants and neuroprotectants in 2003 under patent number 6,630,507.

Why does this matter? This patent essentially acknowledges and affirms the medicinal properties of cannabinoids — the very compounds found in the cannabis plant. It recognizes cannabinoids for their potential in treating specific neurodegenerative diseases, such as Alzheimer's, Parkinson's, and HIV dementia. This is particularly notable because it happened while cannabis remained a Schedule I substance under federal law and Zero Tolerance campaigns were at their peak. This classification not only deems it illegal but also claims that it has a high potential for abuse with "no accepted medical use."

So, on one hand, the government's official stance through the Controlled Substances Act has been that cannabis offers no medicinal benefits. Yet, on the other hand, a governmental body possesses a patent highlighting the therapeutic attributes of the plant's compounds. This duality showcases the layers of interests, contradictions, and complexities inherent in the cannabis prohibition narrative.

Who benefits from this patent? The patent suggests that the government was, at the very least, cognizant of the potential applications of cannabinoids. By securing rights to its medicinal applications, they positioned themselves to capitalize on any future pharmaceutical endeavors leveraging these compounds. This is strikingly contradictory to the overarching narrative that cannabis lacks medicinal properties and has been a point of significant contention among advocates and researchers alike.

This move also raises questions about the role of the pharmaceutical industry. With exclusive rights, the government or any licensed entity could produce cannabinoid-based medications, potentially reaping enormous profits while sidelining the natural, unpatentable plant. All the while, average citizens found themselves facing criminal charges for possessing or consuming the very same compounds that the government deemed beneficial enough to patent. Make it make sense!

This patent exemplifies the tangled web of interests, politics, and profit motives that have clouded the cannabis landscape in the US While advocates and patients face legal hurdles and stigmas, certain entities, including the government itself, maneuver behind the scenes in ways that suggest a deeper understanding and appreciation of the plant's benefits.

The Prison System

Jails, prisons, and correctional facilities (both public and private entities) also benefit from the prohibition of cannabis, as it provides them with a steady stream of inmates who are incarcerated for drug-related offenses. The privatization of prisons has also led to an increase in the number of people being incarcerated for drug offenses, as it is a profitable business for the companies running these institutions.

Jails, prisons, and correctional facilities may benefit from the prohibition of cannabis in several ways:

- *Increased inmate population*: Prohibition of cannabis can result in increased arrests and convictions for drug-related offenses, leading to a larger inmate population. This can translate to increased funding for correctional facilities and job security for corrections staff.
- *Contracted labor*: Many prisons use inmate labor for various tasks such as manufacturing, agriculture, and construction. With more inmates in the system due to drug-related offenses, the facilities can contract more labor and, in turn, increase their revenue.
- *Privatization*: Privately owned prisons may benefit financially from the War on Drugs, as their contracts often stipulate that the state must maintain a certain occupancy rate. This incentivizes the state to maintain a high number of inmates.

The intricate web of prohibition beneficiaries is not simply a matter of law or morality; it is deeply rooted in economic interests, power dynamics, and historical contexts. Various stakeholders, from big agriculture to pharmaceutical giants, from the prison-industrial complex to influential political figures, have found a way to capitalize on the status quo. Their gains often come at the cost of marginalized communities, the stagnation of scientific advancement, and the denial of access to potentially life-changing therapies.

It's essential to recognize that the challenges facing cannabis legalization aren't merely about changing minds over a misunderstood plant. The hurdles are systemic, with a complex network of beneficiaries who have a vested interest in maintaining the current questionable situation. This intricate mosaic of motivations and benefits underscores the depth of the challenge faced by the cannabis industry.

However, understanding this landscape is crucial. In my opinion, by identifying and acknowledging the players and their interests, advocates can strategize more effectively, addressing not just the social and medical arguments for cannabis but the economic and political ones as well. The journey toward legalization and a fair system is full of complex layers. To navigate it effectively, one must be cognizant of all the forces at play, especially those hidden in the shadows of economic gain.

As the push for change continues, it becomes even more vital to be informed and strategic. By understanding the depths of the opposition and its roots, we can hope to pave a way forward that addresses not just the legal status of cannabis but also the broader systemic issues it intertwines with.

Chapter 7
The Promise of Legalization

So far, we've probed deep into the many challenges cannabis faced before emerging as a burgeoning industry. Its rapid ascent as an industry is nothing short of remarkable. The cannabis sector's growth has not only fortified local economies during the pandemic, creating jobs and bolstering government revenues, but has also breathed life into cities previously facing economic hardships. However, it's crucial to note that many markets have been hampered by extreme over-regulation and excessive taxation, making it challenging to establish sustainable business models for operators navigating the government-regulated system. Yet, regardless of these constraints, consumer demand and overall optimistic perception of cannabis in regulated and non-regulated areas have shown a consistent upward trend.

As a longtime advocate in the cannabis sector, I consistently highlight that the push for cannabis reform extends well beyond the plant's recognized medicinal properties. The industry's economic potential is another compelling reason to push for legislative change.

Cannabis enterprises are sprouting up in droves, creating jobs that span from cultivation to manufacturing to administrative and marketing. These roles offer employment to a diverse workforce. This is particularly significant as we are still recovering from the economic ravages of the most recent pandemic.

Having said that, the industry isn't without its challenges. One glaring issue is the exorbitant taxation that cannabis businesses face. This not only makes operations unsustainable but could also backfire on governmental bodies that depend on this revenue. The volatility of the business landscape—here today, gone tomorrow due to sinking in tax debt—means less stability in tax collection, which should be an incentive for governments to reevaluate their taxation strategies.

These tax revenues, ideally, should be reinvested into community services. Some states have channeled these funds into educational programs, infrastructure improvements, and social equity initiatives aimed at mitigating the destructive legacy of cannabis prohibition. However, one thing that stands out to me is the utilization of cannabis tax to increase law enforcement budgets. In my opinion, this raises ethical questions, especially considering the historical context of cannabis criminalization and police involvement.

Speaking from my experience in California's cannabis landscape, the regulatory environment is a work in progress at best. Legislators and policymakers, many of whom are navigating the complexities of cannabis law for the first time, must address a myriad of challenges, including social justice, public health, and market stability. Acknowledging the wrongful criminalization of cannabis opens a Pandora's box of related matters, such as social equity and social justice reform, health and wellness concerns, and youth education. Are any of your city/state/federal officials up for these challenges? I'm sure there aren't many.

Furthermore, there are industry-specific challenges to address, such as market fluctuations, competition from illicit operations, diversity/inclusion, equitable access for individuals who wish to cultivate cannabis at home (after all, it is just a plant!), etc. It's a lot. There is much work to be done to stabilize and legitimize the American cannabis industry fully.

We must admit, despite the human errors and policy missteps, the burgeoning cannabis sector provides a persuasive case study in the broader benefits of drug policy reform. The industry showcases the economic, health, and social advantages that can be realized when we move past archaic laws and unfounded stigmas. For every plant cultivated, dollar made, job opportunity created, tax dollar generated, patient relieved, and nonviolent cannabis offender released from prison, the case for full legalization becomes increasingly undisputable.

Tax Benefits from Cannabis

As per reports from The Washington Post, projections indicate that the legal cannabis industry could generate a massive $131.8 billion in federal tax revenue from 2017 to 2025. Ideally, such income should be funneled toward initiatives that enrich communities, particularly those affected adversely by the War on Drugs.

In numerous Californian cities, a substantial portion of their general fund expenditure is directed toward law enforcement, with police spending accounting for an average of 39% of general fund spending across twenty-eight studied cities. Consequently, without targeted efforts to allocate resources differently, fresh income streams such as cannabis tax revenue that contribute to the general fund disproportionately favor the police departments. One can only hope that the efforts of law enforcement are directed toward stopping cartels and other criminal activity that prevent those navigating the dynamic regulated industry from operating fairly.

Many jurisdictions are deliberately leveraging cannabis revenue to augment their law enforcement budgets. Take my hometown, San Diego, as an example, where priorities have been set to utilize cannabis revenues in enforcing cannabis laws and proactively countering illegal operators. Los Angeles has taken a similar stance, channeling millions of dollars annually from cannabis revenues to a police officer "overtime fund," which is utilized for various law enforcement tasks, including the investigation and enforcement of laws against the illicit market. Meanwhile, the small city of Woodlake, which has a police force of just nine officers and a city police budget of $1.6 million, uses its cannabis revenue to finance an additional officer and other police resources.

On the other hand, there are states like Colorado where things are handled in a more commonsensical manner. The Denver Post highlighted that Colorado utilized $7.3 million from its cannabis tax income on services and housing for the homeless. If the US federal government adopted a similar strategy by regulating cannabis as the state of Colorado and a handful of other states have done, the resulting tax revenue could significantly impact social programs nationwide.

Job Opportunities in the Cannabis Sector

The cannabis industry has emerged as one of the fastest-growing sectors, doubling its size over the past four years and, according to Leafly, a prominent online cannabis resource, creating 121,000 full-time jobs. Forecasts suggest that job growth in the legal cannabis sector will surge by 250 percent in the next decade, outpacing many other industries. In certain states like Massachusetts, the number of cannabis jobs has already overtaken other occupations, such as hairstylists and cosmetologists.

The creation of new jobs as a direct result of the cannabis industry undoubtedly generates enthusiasm and optimism for job seekers, considering the wide range of employment opportunities available. This includes roles such as budtenders/customer service reps, growers, manufacturers, distributors, compliance managers, marketers, accountants, admin, and more.

Reallocating Funds from Prohibition Budgets

According to the American Civil Liberties Union, approximately $7.7 billion is spent annually to enforce the War on Drugs. If cannabis were subjected to a taxation rate comparable to that of tobacco and alcohol, it could potentially generate an estimated annual revenue of $6 billion. A portion of this vast budget can potentially be redirected toward initiatives directly tied to making an impact in the communities affected by the War on Drugs, as well as bolstering cannabis education and improving regulation systems. The redirection of that capital could potentially help disenfranchised communities by the War on Drugs to overcome many pressing challenges.

Given the ineffectiveness of cannabis prohibition and the current American sentiment toward cannabis, there is no justification for such substantial budget allocations. This funding can instead be redirected to remediate the damages to communities that have been disproportionately impacted by harsh prohibition policies. Beyond this, the considerable revenue potential that could be unlocked through federal cannabis reform can stimulate the economy significantly.

The Race to Last Place

As of August 2023, only a few states remain hesitant to address cannabis legalization within their jurisdictions. These states—Idaho, Kansas, Wyoming, and South Carolina—are characterized by conservative political climates and smaller populations, factors that make it difficult to gain widespread support at the ballot box. Additionally, these states have limited resources and are skeptical about the financial gains that could come from a regulated cannabis industry, possibly contributing to their reluctance to join the cannabis regulation arena.

Among these states, Idaho stands out as the most conservative, with a long-standing tradition of conservative politics and rural values. While Kansas and Wyoming also lean conservative, they offer more moderate political pockets and a greater diversity of opinions. Despite these nuances, all four states have generally resisted progressive social and political changes, including cannabis legalization.

Nevertheless, these right-leaning states stand to benefit significantly from legalization as well. Potential gains range from additional tax revenue and job creation to reductions in criminal justice costs and improvements in public health. The tourism sector could also see a boost from the new businesses that a cannabis program could attract.

The degree to which these states would benefit from a regulated cannabis market depends on several factors:

- *Financial Situation:* A state's fiscal health, including budget deficits and revenue needs, could heavily influence the attractiveness of legalization. States with significant budget gaps might find the new tax revenue particularly beneficial.
- *Population Size:* Larger populations could provide a more substantial market for cannabis products, resulting in not just tax revenue but also job opportunities and a platform for social justice initiatives.
- *Political Climate:* States with a supportive political environment and a strong base of advocates are more likely to pass cannabis-friendly legislation, creating a conducive atmosphere for industry growth and community benefits. Regulatory teams well-versed in social equity considerations would be a bonus.
- *Regulatory Structure:* States with reasonable tax policies and business-friendly regulations are more likely to attract investments and foster growth in the regulated cannabis industry.

Most importantly, the path to achieving legalization—and its associated economic and social benefits—is advocacy. Advocacy shapes public opinion and political environments and, by doing so, directly influences the likelihood of achieving policy changes. Activists work to educate the public, raise awareness of the adverse effects of prohibition, and mobilize legalization support. They counter opposition, address concerns, and build coalitions to generate the political will required to enact reform. As such, advocacy remains a potent tool for shaping the ongoing debate around cannabis in the realms of criminal and social justice, healthcare, and economic policy.

Higher Expectations

One thing is for sure: the potential cannabis reform is huge, but as of right now, the regulated cannabis industry is not so business-friendly in the majority of the legal states. The industry seems to be only accessible to those with access to money, social equity programs nationwide have not yielded significant results, the majority of the industry's equity demographic is still rich-white-male, and people continue to be arrested and are currently serving life sentences for nonviolent cannabis offenses. The current laws in most states make it extremely difficult for the average person to start a business. Access to capital is still stifled by the lack of banking opportunities due to the plant's current federal status.

As you must know by now, the cannabis industry is extremely red-tapped and heavily regulated, and the regulations can vary significantly from city to city and state to state. This can create a complex and confusing regulatory landscape that can be difficult for companies of all sizes to navigate. Additionally, the federal ban creates further regulatory challenges for companies operating in states where cannabis is legal due to US IRS Code 280E.

The 280E provision of the Internal Revenue Code disallows cannabis businesses from taking deductions or credits for expenses related to the trafficking of controlled substances. Since cannabis is still illegal at the federal level, cannabis businesses are considered to be "trafficking" a controlled substance and are, therefore, subject to this provision. This means that legal cannabis businesses are unable to deduct expenses such as rent, utilities, wages, and other operating expenses like any other business, leading to a significantly higher tax burden.

As a result, cannabis businesses often face effective tax rates of 70% or more, significantly reducing their profitability and ability to reinvest in their business. This puts cannabis businesses at a disadvantage compared to businesses other industries and makes it difficult for them to operate and expand. It also limits their ability to provide competitive prices and products to consumers.

Limited access to banking and financial services plays a major role in the challenges faced by the industry. Because cannabis is still illegal at the federal level, many banks and financial institutions are hesitant to work with cannabis companies for fear of violating federal laws. This creates a major challenge for the industry, as operators are often unable to access traditional banking services like loans, credit lines, and other forms of financing needed to grow a business.

Without access to these types of financial services, cannabis companies are often forced to rely on cash transactions, which can be risky and inconvenient. Cash is difficult to manage and transport and can also make businesses more vulnerable to theft and other forms of criminal activity. In addition, cash transactions can make it more difficult for businesses to track their finances, which can make it harder to manage costs and plan for the future.

As if all the above weren't enough, without access to traditional financing options, cannabis businesses may struggle to raise the capital they need to expand their operations, develop new products, or invest in new technologies. This can limit their ability to innovate and stay competitive in an increasingly crowded marketplace, making it difficult for them to grow and succeed over the long-term.

Many states' reason to regulate cannabis is the money (a.k.a. tax revenue from regulating the commerce of cannabis). Most of these states have imposed high tax rates on the industry in order to generate revenue and "offset the costs of regulating" it. However, these high tax rates have had a huge negative impact and disastrous consequences for legal cannabis operators, their businesses, and, ultimately, the consumer.

High taxation significantly increases the cost of producing and selling cannabis products, creating another challenge: tough competition with the black market and the growing hemp-derived THC products that have recently flooded all smoke shops throughout the United States. Since illegal operators do not have to pay taxes or comply with regulations, they can often offer products at a lower cost than regulated businesses.

High tax rates can also make it more difficult for legal businesses to attract investment and raise capital. Investors may be hesitant to invest in businesses that face such high tax burdens, as this can limit their potential return on investment and make it more difficult for the business to grow and succeed over the long term.

High tax rates can also create challenges for consumers, as they may have to pay more for legal cannabis products than they would for similar products on the readily available black market. This can make it more difficult for regulated businesses to build a loyal customer base and compete with black and gray market operators who have the capacity to offer more affordable prices.

Beyond the challenges of managing the business, add a new layer of challenges: marketing, promotion, and advertising restrictions. Strict regulations on advertising and marketing continue to plague the cannabis industry despite legalization, under the premise that, as a society, we should prevent overexposure to minors and limit the potential negative effects of cannabis use.

While these regulations are supposed to be implemented for public health and safety, when enforced without a factual basis, they present challenges to the businesses being affected. Despite regulation, cannabis companies are limited in their ability to advertise or market their products through traditional channels like print, radio, and television, which makes it more difficult to reach potential customers, build brand recognition, and create demand.

Additionally, restrictions on advertising and marketing limit the ability of legal businesses to differentiate themselves from the black market. This can put legal businesses at a competitive disadvantage, making it more difficult and costly for them to attract customers, build a loyal customer base, and have at least a legitimate opportunity to pay the high taxes and fees owed to the state in which they operate and to the federal government...yes the feds still collect taxes from a "federally illegal" industry. Riddle me that!

Restrictions on advertising and marketing can also limit the ability of legal businesses to educate consumers about the potential benefits of the cannabis plant, as well as the risks. Without access to effective marketing channels, legal businesses struggle to communicate these messages to consumers, which can create confusion and misunderstanding.

Instagram...which is owned by Meta (previously known as Facebook), has been known to limit the visibility of cannabis content and even delete profiles of content creators and brands that focus on cannabis-related topics. One may assume this is largely because cannabis is still illegal at the federal level and, therefore, falls under the category of "prohibited content" on many social media platforms. But as a person whose businesses have been victims of IG's biased, selective censorship, I assure you they can do better. Cannabis-related content is often flagged or removed by automated systems (a.k.a. algorithms) that are designed to prevent the distribution of prohibited content. These AI systems often make costly mistakes.

Ultimately, these restrictions create significant challenges for cannabis content creators and brands who rely on social media to build their audience and promote their products. Without access to these platforms, it makes it difficult for businesses to reach potential customers, build a loyal following, and advocate for the benefits of the plant. This presents a significant challenge for small businesses and independent creators who may not have the resources to invest in other forms of marketing or advertising.

The inconsistent application of these policies can create confusion and frustration for cannabis-related businesses and content creators. Some accounts may be able to post cannabis-related content without issue, while others may be deleted or limited in their visibility (shadow-banned). This can make it difficult for businesses to build a predictable and reliable social media presence and can create uncertainty around the long-term viability of their marketing strategies.

While social media platforms like Instagram can be an important tool for all businesses and content creators, the restrictions and limitations placed on cannabis-related content create significant challenges for those working in the industry. Finding alternative channels for promotion and marketing while also navigating these restrictions is a key challenge for businesses operating in the legal cannabis industry.

The federal prohibition of cannabis has severely limited the amount of research that can be conducted on the plant and its potential uses. Historically, this has created significant challenges for medical patients, scientists, businesses, and all stakeholders in the space, including those who oppose legalization, as they are deprived of access to the scientific knowledge or data they need to develop a science-backed understanding of the plant and its components.

Without access to this information, companies may be limited in their ability to innovate and stay competitive in the marketplace. This can make it more difficult for them to develop products that meet the needs of consumers, or to identify new areas of growth and opportunity in the industry.

This can make it difficult for legal businesses to differentiate themselves from the black market, as consumers may be wary of using products that have not been thoroughly tested or evaluated. It can also create challenges for legal businesses in terms of regulation and compliance, as they may not have access to the scientific data they need to ensure that their products meet regulatory standards.

The limited access to research caused by the federal prohibition of cannabis is a significant challenge for legal businesses in the industry. Finding ways to access and utilize scientific data and information while also complying with federal regulations is a key challenge for businesses operating in the regulated environment.

Again, the potential of the cannabis industry upon the legalization of the plant at the federal level is huge. The current landscape, with its hurdles and challenges, should not discourage advocates, entrepreneurs, cannabis professionals, consumers, or canna-curious individuals. There is a lot to overcome, but as you read in previous chapters, there is a lot of work that was done by pioneers, and a lot of work is being done as I write these words by innovators. The cannabis collective is making huge waves and strides to be the change and contribute to a future of safe access, research, and fair business. I always like to remind everyone that the industry is still relatively new, and as the legal landscape continues to evolve, many of these challenges are likely to be remediated over time. There is one thing we all can agree upon: maximizing the potential of the plant is something worth looking forward to.

Chapter 8

Is the Grass Truly Greener?

Potential Adverse Effects of Legalization

The journey toward cannabis legalization is marked by a mix of positives and hurdles. While the promise of economic, social, and health benefits is significant, it's crucial to navigate a few key challenges to ensure these advantages fully materialize without unwanted side effects. Among these challenges are the potential for economic gains to fall short of expectations, the complexity of regulations for local authorities and cannabis enterprises, environmental concerns, and issues related to public health and safety. Moreover, the hoped-for progress in social and racial justice may not be as substantial as many advocates would like.

Support for cannabis legalization among American adults has seen a remarkable increase over the years, jumping from 12% in 1969 to nearly 70% in 2020, reflecting a significant shift in public opinion. This shift was further highlighted during the COVID-19 pandemic when numerous state and local governments deemed cannabis services essential, underscoring its growing acceptance and integration into mainstream society.

Child Safety in the Era of Cannabis Legalization

As cannabis legalization gains momentum across the United States, one of the growing concerns is the unintentional exposure of children to cannabis products. While adult consumption continues working itself toward normalization, the complexities surrounding safe storage, appropriate packaging, and public education have not kept pace with the speed of legalization.

One reason for this is the advent of edible cannabis products that often resemble candies, chocolates, or baked goods. Many edibles may be particularly appealing to children and can easily be mistaken for "regular" food items, even by adults. The danger here lies not just in the immediate effects of THC, which is the psychoactive component of cannabis, but also in the possibility of consuming a dangerously high dosage. This can lead to a range of symptoms, from dizziness and confusion to more severe consequences, such as impaired motor functions, similar to being drunk.

There have been reports of increased emergency room visits related to unintentional cannabis exposure in children. A study published in *The Journal of Pediatrics* found that emergency department visits and regional poison center calls for pediatric cannabis cases increased significantly in states that had legalized it. Moreover, states that had more relaxed restrictions on cannabis had higher rates of unintentional exposure among children compared to states with more stringent controls.

Some steps have been taken to address this issue, including the introduction of child-resistant packaging and warning labels. However, there is still much to be done in terms of public implementation of education and regulation. It is imperative for parents and caregivers to be intentional about storing cannabis and to remain informed about the risks associated with cannabis products around children, similar to the education about prescription medications or household cleaning agents that could be harmful if ingested.

State agencies and cannabis producers have a role to play in this regard. Just as alcohol and tobacco products come with age restrictions and warning labels, cannabis is also subject to stringent safety measures to prevent accidental ingestion. This includes standardized child-proof packaging for edibles, public service announcements targeting parents, and perhaps even including safety locks on products meant for home use.

It's important to highlight that edibles aren't exclusively purchased from stores; they can also be homemade. Not too long ago, a friend and I baked cannabis-infused chocolate chip cookies each had an estimated 40 mg of THC. After baking, I placed them in a cookie jar on my kitchen counter. While I don't have kids, an incident occurred involving an adult, Candy, who oversees my weekly housekeeping. While I wasn't at home, she unknowingly consumed two of these cookies. Later that day, I found out her daughter had to rush her to the hospital, mistaking her symptoms for a stroke. At the hospital, Candy discovered her unexpected high was due to cannabis, which I confirmed were the cookies she ate at my home. Hence, the accidental consumption of cannabis isn't just a concern for children; adults and even pets can be affected too.

As cannabis legalization and its normalization in society progress, incidents like these could become more common. Despite there being no documented cases of fatalities from cannabis overdose, the risk of accidental ingestion poses a realistic safety concern. The experience of Candy, who unwittingly ate cannabis-infused cookies, underscores that adults are also at risk. It highlights the need for caution and awareness around edible cannabis products, especially in environments where individuals might not expect to encounter them.

One more thing I want to add on this topic for transparency purposes is that the study published in *The Journal of Pediatrics* did not differentiate between homemade cannabis-infused edibles and edibles purchased at a cannabis retailer. Furthermore, the study did not differentiate between regulated edibles and black-market products. Either way, the moral of the story is this: parents (including fur-baby parents), caretakers, and adults should be mindful of how and where we store our cannabis products, and we also need to be stern in educating children about the risks.

Understanding Cannabinoid Hyperemesis Syndrome

Another potential consideration is the rise of a condition called Cannabinoid Hyperemesis Syndrome (CHS). This relatively rare but increasingly documented condition is characterized by cyclic episodes of nausea and vomiting after consuming cannabis. CHS has puzzled healthcare providers since its identification, largely because cannabis has been traditionally associated with the alleviation of nausea and vomiting rather than the induction of these symptoms.

CHS is typically seen in long-term, heavy cannabis consumers, and the syndrome's symptoms often lead to repeated emergency room visits, with patients usually receiving a wide range of gastrointestinal and psychotropic medications to little avail. The most effective treatment for CHS appears to be the cessation of cannabis use, but it appears that diagnosis may be tricky, as patients may be reluctant to disclose their cannabis use to healthcare providers. In addition, many medical professionals remain unaware of the condition due to its relatively recent identification and the prevailing notion of cannabis as an antiemetic.

Why CHS occurs remains an area of active research, but some theories suggest it could be related to the disruption of the endocannabinoid system in the gut, brain, and liver, where cannabis receptors are found. Another hypothesis is that the excessive accumulation of cannabinoids with long-term frequent use may cause a toxic effect, leading to CHS symptoms in some cases.

The commercialization of cannabis products has led to greater potency and availability. Public awareness of the syndrome remains relatively low, even among frequent cannabis users, given that cannabis is increasingly seen as a lifestyle wellness product. As cannabis becomes more integrated into medical and recreational settings, healthcare systems will need to adapt and educate both providers and the public about the full range of cannabis-related health outcomes, both positive and negative. CHS serves as a cautionary example that with greater access to cannabis comes the responsibility to understand its effects on health.

Detecting Cannabis Impairment

The complexities surrounding cannabis and certain employment areas create a layered challenge, one that impacts individuals, organizations, and regulatory entities. As cannabis continues to gain recognition as a legitimate form of medicine for many, these intricacies become even more apparent, prompting a closer examination of how the plant intersects with the workplace.

Cannabis is, without a doubt, a form of medicine for countless individuals. The stories of people finding relief and improved function through cannabis are both numerous and compelling. One need only search "cannabis and tremors" on YouTube to discover a plethora of firsthand accounts. Take, for instance, the story of Norma, who battled Dystonia for seventeen years. Dystonia is a neurological movement disorder characterized by involuntary (unintended) muscle contractions that cause slow, repetitive movements or abnormal postures that can sometimes be painful. Through the use of CBD, a cannabinoid derived from cannabis, she found relief and a renewed lease on life. While Norma may be a stranger, her story is just one of countless others.

Personally, I can attest to the transformative power of cannabis. A traumatic brain injury I sustained during my service in the US Navy left me grappling with severe sleep disturbances. The transition to civilian life only exacerbated this issue. Cannabis became a lifeline, enabling me to manage my condition and cope with the consequences of sleep deprivation. My experience is just one of many, a testament to the diverse ways in which cannabis medicine can positively impact individuals.

Yet, cannabis is not a one-size-fits-all solution. While some find solace and relief, others have reported experiencing anxiety, paranoia, and other symptoms. The profoundly personal nature of these experiences emphasizes the importance of understanding and managing cannabis use in the context of public safety.

Navigating this complex landscape is indeed challenging. As cannabis legalization continues to evolve, it becomes increasingly crucial to strike a balance that accommodates the therapeutic needs of individuals while safeguarding workplace integrity and public safety. Finding a solution that respects the deeply personal nature of cannabis experiences and ensures responsible use is a pressing concern. It's a testament to the intricate dance between personal freedom, medical necessity, and societal responsibility in the ever-evolving world of cannabis.

Furthermore, the limitations of current methods for determining cannabis impairment only add another complexity layer to the issue. While lab testing for THC in the blood is the standard procedure for ascertaining cannabis use, it's far from a perfect system. The main issue lies in the fact that levels of THC in the blood are not reliable indicators of impairment. Unlike alcohol, where a certain blood concentration level has been universally accepted as a measure of impairment, THC doesn't work in the same way. For habitual users, high levels of THC might be present in the blood without any signs of impairment. Additionally, trace amounts of THC can remain in the blood long after the effects have worn off, making it an unreliable indicator of present impairment.

I believe the current methods for detecting cannabis exposure place medical cannabis patients at a disadvantage. Patients may require cannabis for the treatment of various conditions but may find themselves at risk of disciplinary action at the workplace due to THC showing up in drug tests. This scenario illustrates the urgent need for more refined methodologies that can accurately measure not just cannabis exposure but also its associated impairment, if any.

In the face of these challenges, efforts are underway to improve the technology used to detect cannabis impairment. Companies are in the process of developing breathalyzer devices, although these are currently designed to only measure exposure, not impairment. One can only hope that the goal of these ongoing initiatives is to create a standard that can provide a reliable measure of functional impairment without penalizing those who have legally consumed cannabis for medical reasons.

As the legal landscape for cannabis continues to develop, so too must our methods for responsibly managing its use in various societal contexts, including the workplace. Without accurate, reliable measures for cannabis impairment, we risk creating policies that unfairly penalize users without effectively addressing the issues at hand. The development of better detection methods is not just a scientific challenge but also a potential necessity as we aim for a more nuanced and equitable approach to cannabis legalization and its subsequent impact on the workplace.

Hemp-Derived THC vs. Cannabis THC

The emergence of hemp-derived THC, specifically Delta-9 THC, has introduced a significant curveball into the cannabis landscape, raising questions about its legal status and creating challenges for law enforcement and consumer safety.

As mentioned in an earlier chapter, in 2018, the US legalized hemp, a variety of the cannabis plant that contains 0.3% or less of Delta-9 THC, the psychoactive compound responsible for the "high" associated with marijuana consumption. This distinction was intended to support struggling farmers by allowing them to cultivate industrial hemp and enabled the interstate sale of CBD, resulting in the explosive growth of a multibillion-dollar industry.

Delta-9 THC is the most well-known variant of tetrahydrocannabinol, commonly referred to as THC, and is the compound classified as a Schedule I drug and subject to legal potency limits in hemp plants. Regardless of its source, Delta-9 THC behaves the same way in the body, binding to cannabinoid receptors and producing the euphoric effects when consumed.

Hemp-derived Delta-9 THC is typically produced using one of two methods: extraction directly from the hemp plant or by chemical conversion of CBD from hemp into THC by cyclization (the closure of a ring after an acid-catalyzed activation of a double bond) (Marzullo et al. 2020). Some manufacturers have exploited regulatory gaps, particularly regarding the calculation of THC content on a "dry-weight basis" for various products like oils and edibles, allowing them to bypass federal potency limits.

Hemp Delta-9 products have cleverly navigated the Farm Bill's 0.3% THC limit by dry weight. This means a 10g gummy could contain up to 30mg of Delta-9 THC and still comply with legal standards. This is in stark contrast to the Schedule 1 subjected-cannabis edibles found in legal states such as California and Colorado, where servings typically contain only 5mg or 10mg of Delta-9 THC. As a direct result of the current legal wording, intoxicating hemp-based Delta-9 THC products have become widely accessible in most states, illustrating a loophole that allows for higher THC levels than many regulated cannabis products.

Relying on the loophole and hemp's legal status, manufacturers and brands in the hemp industry see an opportunity to sell Delta-9 THC products outside licensed dispensaries in states where cannabis is legal and beyond. Regulated dispensaries are often subject to stringent regulations and high taxes, resulting in narrower profit margins. Consequently, sellers have been drawn to CBD stores, smoke shops, grocery stores, bars, and other retail outlets to market seemingly identical products labeled as hemp-derived Delta-9 THC. An April study from CBD Oracle reported that approximately 120 brands are selling such products online.

However, a significant red flag has emerged with many so-called "hemp-derived" Delta-9 THC products. Laboratory analyses conducted on fifty-three such products revealed that over a quarter contained THC derived from traditional cannabis plants, not hemp. Additionally, nearly half of the products contained THC that had been chemically converted from CBD rather than being naturally derived from hemp. Only a minority, approximately 18.4%, likely used genuinely hemp-derived Delta-9 THC.

This situation raises concerns about product quality, consistency, and safety. The lack of regulation surrounding the synthesis of Delta-9 THC, Delta-8 THC, THC-O, and other psychoactive cannabinoids further complicates the issue. As the industry continues to make strides, addressing these challenges becomes paramount to ensuring consumer safety and compliance.

The DEA and Cannabis in the Twenty-first Century

Despite notable progress in cannabis legalization at the state level, the realm of federal oversight remains a complex and evolving area, often generating perplexing circumstances for the budding space. One such example is the DEA's issuance of licenses for medical cannabis research, a move that appears to signify a step forward for scientific exploration but simultaneously underscores the current federal status of cannabis as a controlled substance. This duality poses a considerable conflict of interest for businesses navigating the regulated industry, consumers all over the country, and most importantly, those who are still incarcerated for cannabis.

The DEA's policy aims to facilitate research involving cannabis and its various chemical components. According to their website, the DEA seeks to increase the number of entities registered under the CSA to cultivate cannabis, thereby ensuring a more robust supply of "research-grade" cannabis for private and public researchers across the United States. This policy marks a significant turn in how the DEA evaluates applications for registration, aligning them with the CSA and the United States' obligations under international drug control treaties.

For nearly half a century, the United States has relied on a single grower operating under a contract with the National Institute on Drug Abuse (NIDA) to produce cannabis for research purposes. This arrangement was historically perceived as the most suitable method to fulfill the country's obligations under international drug control treaties. However, as public interest in cannabis-related research, particularly regarding cannabinoids, has surged in recent years, the limitations of this single-grower system have become very evident.

The traditional system primarily catered to the needs of federally funded research, with no established pathway for commercial entities to develop cannabis-based products legally. In contrast, the new approach outlined in this policy statement permits individuals and organizations to register with the DEA to cultivate the plant, not only for research but also for commercial ventures funded by the private sector, focusing on product development. Furthermore, this approach allows pharmaceutical firms to legally produce cannabis-derived drugs should scientific knowledge advance and demonstrate their efficacy for medical use. The latter is a huge red flag and creates an element of skepticism surrounding the DEA's program. It appears that the historically prohibitionist law enforcement organization is establishing a federal framework tailored toward pharmaceutical interests. Notably, the US government held patents on certain cannabinoids for two decades, licensing them to select pharmaceutical companies. Under these agreements, if these companies develop successful drugs from these patented materials, the National Institutes of Health (NIH) receives a portion of the sales as royalties.

Not the federal government profiting from the sale of drugs derived from specific cannabinoids after over 100 years of prohibition... For instance, GW Pharmaceuticals created the epilepsy medication Epidiolex using cannabinoids patented by the NIH. Epidiolex could generate annual revenues exceeding $2 billion, with the NIH benefiting from royalties on each sale. Currently, the NIH holds over 4,000 patents, with ninety-three of them contributing to the development of 34 FDA-approved drugs, generating nearly $2 billion in revenue.

These complexities raise questions about the intersection of federal oversight, pharmaceutical interests, and the growing cannabis sector. As we navigate this intricate landscape, it becomes increasingly important to understand how these factors may impact the future of cannabis research, product development, and accessibility.

Evolution of Potency

In the world of cannabis, a significant transformation has occurred in recent years that calls for our attention. Even though modern cannabis enthusiasts have access to astonishingly high THC levels, this was far from the norm in the past. Over time, the THC content in cannabis has seen a substantial increase, primarily due to more methodical breeding techniques. In fact, the most potent strains found in today's dispensaries are several times stronger than the best cannabis available fifty years ago. Consequently, the surge in THC concentrations in cannabis products raises valid concerns, especially for those new to its consumption or individuals susceptible to mental health challenges. These concerns undoubtedly fall within the realm of public health.

As Deepak Cyril D'Souza, MD, the Albert E Kent Professor of Psychiatry at Yale School of Medicine, aptly puts it, "The marijuana and cannabis products that your grandparents may have used are very different from what's out there now."

Over the past few decades, the THC content in cannabis has undergone a remarkable transformation. In 1995, the average THC content in cannabis confiscated by the Drug Enforcement Administration hovered around 4%. Fast forward to 2017, and that figure had skyrocketed to 17%, with the trend continuing upward. Beyond the traditional plant form, an array of cannabis products boasting even higher THC concentrations, such as dabs, oils, and edibles, are readily available, with some reaching levels as high as 90%.

At this very moment, I am getting ready to roll a joint from California's brand Cannabiotix Heirbloom Legacy Flower. The cultivar is a sativa-leaning Super Silver Haze with a potency of 23.42%...But I digress.

In the United States, cannabis cultivation has, for the most part, zeroed in on THC over the past half-century. In the early days of cannabis breeding, THC levels were minuscule by today's standards. In fact, during the 1970s, average THC levels remained just below 5% (sometimes even lower, contingent on the cannabis quality). Given

THC's central role in producing the sought-after psychoactive effects, high-THC cannabis has always been in demand. As with any market driven by demand, supply responds accordingly. To meet the growing appetite for THC, cannabis breeding has evolved into a sophisticated science, spanning decades of dedicated cultivation.

Throughout the late twentieth and early twenty-first centuries, purposeful cannabis breeding has yielded some exceptionally high-THC strains/cultivars that are now accessible to consumers.

Contemporary cannabis research extends beyond individual cannabinoids, emphasizing the interactions among different compounds. While THC and CBD undoubtedly influence the overall cannabis experience, the "entourage effect," driven by the interplay of multiple compounds, significantly contributes to the distinct characteristics of a particular cannabis cultivar.

Today, the cannabis industry is increasingly focused on exploring new cannabinoids and other components of the cannabis flower, including terpenoids, sterols, and flavonoids. Their "entourage effect" offers unique effects, and a thorough understanding of a strain's total cannabinoid content (TAC) provides consumers with predictability. For example, cannabinoids like CBG may offer relief from pain, while CBN is recognized for its sleep-inducing properties. As the industry shifts away from a singular focus on THC, customers can expect more tailored cannabis products that cater to their specific needs, promising a more controlled and personalized experience.

Natural vs. Synthetic Terpenes

The olfactory delight of cannabis flower, often accompanied by an explosion of colors, owes much of its charm to the presence of terpenoids, commonly known as terpenes. These terpenoids are secreted within the same trichome glands that produce cannabinoids like cannabigerol or cannabidiol. While naturally derived botanical terpenes are celebrated for their soothing effects on the body and mind, a new player has entered the cannabis scene: synthetic terpenes. But with this innovation comes an important question: Are synthetic terpenes safe for us?

It is not uncommon for cannabis manufacturers to incorporate added terpenes into oils, tinctures, ointments, beverages, and edibles with the aim of enhancing the overall experience or specific health benefits of cannabis-based products. Researchers are diving deeper into the individual properties of terpenes, such as linalool, a terpene also found in lavender known for its anti-anxiety effects. While this research is promising, the intricate interplay between different terpenoids and cannabinoids remains a less-explored territory.

Botanical terpenes, naturally produced by the plant, serve a dual purpose: protecting the plant from predators and attracting pollinators. Within the vast array of cannabis strains, various chemical varieties, often referred to as chemovars, exist, each boasting its unique signature of terpenes and cannabinoids. For instance, the Gelato strain is renowned for its high Caryophyllene, Limonene, and Linalool content, which collectively impart anti-inflammatory, energetic, and relaxing effects. Interestingly, cannabis-based products made from Gelato flower may have varying chemical compositions.

As demand for terpenoids surges, we can anticipate a rise in terpene content. Many consumers are discerning, and terpenes often drive their strain preferences. Consequently, synthetic terpenes are gaining ground too.

Plant-derived terpenes are extracted from the plant before undergoing distillation, preserving their potency. For instance, "live" resin is created by flash-freezing buds to retain terpene content, as high heat can denature them.

Terpenes share the same chemical makeup across nature, as seen with myrcene in thyme and mango, which is identical to the myrcene found in the Blue Dream cannabis flower. Both are considered botanical terpenes. A slight distinction exists between botanical and synthetic terpenes, with the former akin to organic and the latter to genetically modified organism (GMO) products. Synthetic terpenoids are produced in a lab through chemical blending and manipulation, offering the possibility of the genetically modified creation of a customized terpene profile.

Synthetic terpenes are known for their heightened aromas and flavors due to higher concentrations. Although they hold potential for customizable terpene profiles, more research is required to comprehend how synthetic and natural terpenes interact, both with each other and within the body.

The production of synthetic terpenes involves processes like dilution, re-distillation, and reconstruction. While botanical terpenoids typically maintain the naturally occurring properties cannabis consumers seek, synthetic terpenes might employ chemicals to mimic these characteristics.

One major issue arises when companies falsely market products containing synthetic terpenes as "all-natural." As consumers become more informed, they demand transparency regarding the source of terpenes in their cannabinoid products, along with the inclusion of essential oils. While synthetic terpenes may eventually prove to be safe, their long-term effects and the potential residues left behind by these synthetics remain unknown. As with GMO products, a level of caution is warranted when considering the use of synthetic terpenes.

A Resilient Black Market

Despite the legalization of cannabis in various states, the illegal market for this beloved plant continues to thrive. In some cases, it's even more active than it has been in years. California, a state often at the forefront of progressive policies, legalized cannabis with grand ambitions. The intent was clear: bring marijuana out of the shadows, eliminate the illegal market, and establish a regulated, taxed industry. However, behind the scenes of the Golden State's industry lies a web of challenges and a relentless black market.

In just the past year, California has witnessed several massive illegal cannabis busts. Authorities confiscated a staggering 20 tons of cannabis from a series of illicit farms, stumbled upon $8 million worth of plants hidden in a seemingly abandoned warehouse next to a busy highway, and cracked down on over 100 illegal operations in the southern town of Anza just a few months ago.

Proposition 64, the 2016 initiative that set the wheels of legalization in motion, had noble goals. It aimed to shift cannabis production and sales away from the black market, replacing it with a legal, regulated framework designed to provide access to the plant, access to business opportunities within the industry, and generate tax revenue for the state and local municipalities.

Yet, we find ourselves falling short of these voter-mandated objectives, and much of the cannabis industry's challenges can be traced back to two critical flaws in Prop. 64: exorbitant taxes and local control.

Consider this stark comparison: the state excise tax on a bottle of wine is a mere four cents. In contrast, an eighth ounce of cannabis is subjected to a staggering $4.90 in taxes, over 100 times higher. This is further compounded by numerous local taxes applied at each stage of the supply chain, from cultivation to manufacturing, distribution, and retail. Some areas even impose a "road tax" for transportation.

California is not alone in grappling with taxation challenges. Colorado, Oregon, and Washington all impose substantial taxes, creating opportunities for illegal operations to flourish as their prices are more appealing to the consumer. Moreover, illegal businesses have become more prominent in legalized states, as some choose to operate without a legal license while presenting themselves as licensed dealers. Many consumers cannot tell the difference.

What is the result for legal/regulated operators? An aggregate tax burden that often exceeds 50% of the product's original price. Far from driving out the illicit market, these taxes create an environment where illegal cannabis can thrive. Without substantial tax reforms, the battle against illegal cannabis remains an uphill struggle.

The second major flaw lies in the requirement for cannabis businesses to obtain permits from both local jurisdictions and the state. While this might seem reasonable, it has led to widespread bans on cannabis in many areas. This has effectively handed two-thirds of the market back to the black market.

In these regions, unregulated, untaxed, and untested cannabis continues to dominate, as consumers are left with limited options. California's cannabis industry, like its counterparts in wine, technology, and entertainment, should be a thriving heritage sector supported by thoughtful legislation and regulation.

To realize this potential, immediate changes are necessary. Access to legal cannabis must become easier and more affordable for consumers, but it starts at the regulatory level. Cannabis regulations must be business friendly. Until then, the bulk of the industry will remain in the shadows as legacy operators will logically remain operating in the black market, cartels will continue to fuel their operations, and legal businesses will continue to be short-lived due to the unstable and unreasonable business environment in the regulated world.

Environmental Impact

Despite its reputation for environmental consciousness, the cannabis industry grapples with significant environmental challenges. Legalization has ushered in a burgeoning industry, but it has also revealed pressing environmental concerns that demand our attention.

Despite the cannabis industry not yet reaching its full potential, it's exciting to see new businesses and brands entering the scene daily, bringing a variety of innovative concepts, products, and services. However, this rapid influx of newcomers poses a challenge in terms of sustainability. Given that cannabis isn't federally legal and lacks standardized practices for its cultivation, production, and distribution, there's a pressing need to spotlight these issues. It's crucial for both consumers and businesses involved with cannabis retailers to be aware of and address these growing pains as the industry continues to evolve.

Cannabis cultivation comes in three primary forms: indoor, outdoor, and greenhouse setups, each with its unique methodology and challenges. Commercial outdoor growing is the most traditional form, using large land areas for cultivation. Greenhouses frequently blend indoor and outdoor techniques, manipulating light exposure with covers to control the plant life cycle. Indoor cultivation allows for precise control over the environment, often leading to higher quality and yields but at the cost of significant energy use and waste. Notably, the energy costs vary drastically across these methods, with outdoor growing being the most energy-efficient and least carbon-intensive option.

The push toward outdoor cultivation is also fueled by the growing market for processed cannabis products, which can mitigate the quality variances of outdoor-grown cannabis. However, regulatory barriers often restrict outdoor cultivation, forcing many to choose indoor setups that have higher electricity demands by default. State laws, like those in Illinois, may outright ban outdoor cultivation, while others impose strict regulations.

Environmental concerns are becoming increasingly significant, with cross-pollination issues between cannabis and hemp plants threatening crop yields and quality. Initiatives like Colorado's working group and research funded by the USDA aim to address these challenges, emphasizing the importance of supporting outdoor cultivation to reduce the industry's energy consumption and carbon footprint. Encouraging outdoor cultivation through regulatory reform and incentives could significantly improve the sustainability of cannabis cultivation, highlighting the need for policy reform that supports environmental objectives.

Soil Degradation and Remediation

Like conventional agriculture, cannabis cultivation can lead to soil degradation, endangering a crucial component of the ecosystem. Soil erosion, loss of nutrients, decreased organic carbon content, and heightened soil acidity are all consequences associated with destructive agricultural practices. However, if regulation is based on embracing eco-friendly practices, it can serve as a model for mitigating the environmental degradation and climate change impacts prevalent in traditional agriculture.

Furthermore, the cannabis industry can also play a role in environmental remediation. Industrial hemp has the remarkable ability to absorb harmful contaminants, including radioactive materials and heavy metals, from the soil. To ensure safety, soils must undergo rigorous and regular quality testing, and any potential flower from hemp plants intended for remediation purposes should never be consumed.

When cultivators lean on chemical pesticides and other synthetic enhancers to boost their yields, they inadvertently weaken the soil and disrupt its ecological harmony. To counteract this, adopting sustainable and regenerative farming practices is crucial. Sustainable cultivation ensures we safeguard our precious resources for the future without compromising on our present requirements. Meanwhile, regenerative techniques, including employing practices like composting and no-till farming, take it a step further by enriching the soil, revitalizing its nutrients, and enhancing biodiversity. These methods not only nurture the soil but also contribute to a healthier ecosystem overall.

Balancing Thirst with Responsibility

Cannabis cultivation, like many other crops, often relies on artificial irrigation, which can strain water resources and pose environmental risks. Agricultural runoff from cannabis and non-cannabis farming introduces pollutants, including pesticides, heavy metals, and excess nutrients, into ecosystems. Indoor cultivation, while efficient, can stress municipal water systems by discharging excess nutrients and industrial cleaners, leading to increased carbon emissions and indirect air quality consequences.

Water theft and diversions, particularly by unauthorized cannabis growers, pose a significant problem in drought-affected states like California, Oregon, and Nevada. Nevada alone has an estimated 3,500 to 4,000 illegal growers. A study by the Illinois Valley Soil and Water

Conservation District highlighted that in 2021, unlicensed cultivators in the Illinois Valley consumed around 414 million gallons of water.

This issue extends to states like California, where illegal cultivation on public lands is widespread. Greta Wengert, the executive director of the Integral Ecology Research Center, points out that these illicit sites divert billions of gallons of water annually for their operations. This not only constitutes water theft but also deprives the public and local wildlife of crucial water resources.

Lighting the Way to Sustainability

The cannabis industry's diverse cultivation and production environments demand various energy infrastructures, some of which can be energy intensive. Innovations in energy-efficient practices can reduce greenhouse gas emissions stemming from power generation. Efficient data collection is a crucial first step in identifying methods to reduce fossil fuel consumption and enhance energy efficiency at individual facilities.

Industrial-scale cannabis cultivation and processing generate significant waste, comprising organic plant waste and single-use consumer packaging. Inefficient waste management practices contribute to environmental problems, including excessive landfilling, ocean pollution, and greenhouse gas emissions. Single-use vape pen cartridges, disposable plastic containers, and excessive packaging add to the environmental burden.

As a burgeoning industry, the cannabis sector has the opportunity to lead by example, setting a high standard for sustainable practices. Businesses that embrace environmental sustainability can reduce their ecological footprint while boosting profits and offering cost savings to consumers. Collaborative efforts between government bodies and the industry to establish supportive resources, regulations, and policies are vital for achieving these goals. Striving for cooperative policies and standards across local, state, regional, and national levels is imperative for the sustainable evolution of cannabis commerce.

Chapter 9
Terms Matter

Cannabis vs. Marijuana

I use the terms "cannabis" and "marijuana" alternatively with a personal bias, although without any specific basis. I often use "cannabis" to refer to the plant (Cannabis sativa or C. indica) or the industry and "marijuana" when making reference to the cultural aspects of the space. I have observed many people maintain the distinction between the two terms.

This preference, however, hides a dispute I think should be addressed. A significant portion of individuals, particularly among cannabis advocates, reject the term "marijuana" in favor of "cannabis." Those opposing the term "marijuana" argue that it's historically racialized (marihuana), propagated by scholars, government officials, and media to sway public sentiment against both the substance and certain demographic groups. There is plenty of historical basis to support this claim.

In the United States' history, aspects such as words, music, products, and behaviors have been tagged in manners that overtly or subtly introduce race in their usage. This racialization of language has impacted African Americans and immigrants from Latin America, Asia, Ireland, Italy, Eastern Europe, and beyond.

The term "marijuana" (also "marihuana") originates from Mexican Spanish, used in the early twentieth century as a slang term for cannabis. Yet, during and after the Spanish-American War, American animosity toward Mexicans and Mexican immigrants escalated. Tensions were particularly intense along the US's southern border, leading to widespread vilification of these groups through media, entertainment, and political rhetoric. "Marijuana" became popular in the 1930s in the US as prohibition supporters exploited prejudice against marginalized minority groups, especially Mexican immigrants.

As the influx of Mexican immigrants increased, Americans' discomfort grew. Stereotypes, including "Mexicans using marihuana," were used to blame these newcomers for societal problems, such as petty crime and disturbances. Media reports began echoing these stereotypes, marking a striking change in the language surrounding "marijuana."

This linguistic battle extended beyond the media and into official terminology. Government officials like Harry Anslinger, head of the Federal Bureau of Narcotics from 1930 to 1962, gladly partook. Known for his hardline stance on drug prohibition and evident racism, Anslinger fervently adopted "marihuana" in his anti-drug crusade. He exploited the term's associations with Mexico to further his objectives. In one of his essays, Anslinger discussed the introduction of marijuana in the US and its impacts, painting it as a terrifying, crime-inducing substance.

Alongside Anslinger, local law enforcement chiefs and district attorneys played a significant part in not only popularizing the term "marijuana" but also smearing it with racial bias. These government officials' endeavors were blatant in their objective: to associate marijuana with foreign, unfamiliar, or feared demographics and to tie its usage to lawlessness and severe criminal acts. In essence, marijuana—not cannabis or hemp—was painted as a societal menace introduced by those we fear or should fear. The racial instigation was clear, and "marijuana" became the term of choice for those delivering xenophobic narratives.

The refusal to use "marijuana" by the advocacy community is based on a valid understanding of the term's historical application. Authors and speakers who favor "cannabis" are entirely justified.

Let's discuss other terms and concepts of major importance in cannabis. Understanding these terms is essential for both novice and experienced cannabis stakeholders, as they provide the necessary context for understanding the industry, the plant's uses, effects, culture, and regulation.

Drug Policy Reform

Drug Policy Reform is a broad term that covers the movement to change policies that inhibit access to and use of drugs, including cannabis, and shift the focus from punishment to public health. Ideally, Drug Policy Reform should help to redress the negative consequences of drug prohibition and criminalization by proposing better ways to rectify stigmatization, over-incarceration, and infringed civil liberties with the purpose of effectively reducing drug use and improving public safety.

Drug policy reform advocacy places emphasis on a variety of strategies:

- *Decriminalization:* This involves reducing or removing criminal penalties for the possession and use of small amounts of drugs. It is aimed at preventing the detrimental lifelong consequences of criminal records for drug users who are otherwise law-abiding citizens. Portugal is often cited as a successful example of drug decriminalization, where drug use is treated as a public health rather than a criminal issue.
- *Legalization and Regulation:* This approach goes a step further by making the sale and use of a substance legal under a

regulated system. This has been the trend for cannabis in many US states and countries like Canada and Uruguay. Legalization ensures quality control, undermines black-market trade, and allows for tax revenue generation from sales.

- *Harm Reduction:* This strategy acknowledges that drug use is a part of our society and focuses on minimizing its harm without criminalizing its use. Policies may include needle-exchange programs, supervised consumption facilities, or providing access to naloxone to prevent opioid overdose deaths.

- *Access to Treatment:* Advocates for drug policy reform often push for better access to rehabilitation services and for treating drug use as a public health issue rather than a criminal one. This could mean increased funding for treatment centers or policies that favor treatment over incarceration.

- *Social Justice:* Many advocates focus on addressing racial and social inequities in drug law enforcement, given the disproportionate impact of drug prohibition on marginalized communities. This includes advocacy for cannabis equity programs, which aim to ensure that those most harmed by the War on Drugs have an opportunity to participate in the legal cannabis industry.

Drug policy reform is a multifaceted movement that goes beyond simply legalizing drugs; it involves changing societal attitudes, reforming punitive laws, and adopting a more holistic, health-focused approach to drug use.

Legalization vs. Decriminalization

The topic of legalizing and decriminalizing cannabis has sparked a lot of controversy in the United States in the past four decades. While certain states have legalized the plant for medical use, some, like Colorado, Washington, California, and New York, have even gone as far as to legalize the adult or recreational use of the plant. In several cities, municipalities, and states, lawmakers propose decriminalization measures to be included on their upcoming ballots.

It's important to note that the terms "legalization" and "decriminalization" are often used interchangeably, but they have distinct meanings. As the debate rages on, it's crucial to understand the nuanced differences between these two approaches to drug policy as they both have different implications and outcomes.

Here's how they compare and contrast:

- *Definition:* Cannabis legalization refers to the process of making cannabis use, possession, and sale legal under certain conditions, while cannabis decriminalization refers to the process of reducing or eliminating criminal penalties for cannabis use and possession.
- *Legal status:* Legalization makes cannabis fully legal and regulated, whereas decriminalization usually means that cannabis possession and use remain illegal but are treated as minor offenses and subject to civil fines rather than criminal penalties.
- *Availability:* Legalization makes cannabis widely available through licensed dispensaries and retailers. While decriminalization does not necessarily increase availability, it may reduce the risk of arrest and imprisonment for minor cannabis-related offenses.
- *Regulation:* Legalization typically involves regulations on production, distribution, and sale of cannabis, including age restrictions, quality control, and licensing requirements, while decriminalization does not necessarily include regulations, but may allow for personal use and possession without criminal penalties.

- *Taxation:* Legalization typically involves taxation on cannabis sales, which generates revenue for the government, whereas decriminalization does not generate significant revenue.
- *Impact on criminal justice:* Legalization reduces the number of arrests, prosecutions, and incarcerations related to cannabis, while decriminalization reduces the severity of penalties for minor cannabis offenses but may not necessarily reduce the number of arrests and prosecutions.
- *Public health implications:* Legalization allows for the regulation and control of cannabis production and distribution, which may reduce the risks associated with unregulated cannabis use, whereas decriminalization does not necessarily address public health concerns related to cannabis use.

Cannabis legalization and decriminalization represent different approaches to addressing the negative consequences of cannabis prohibition, and each has its own advantages and drawbacks. Legalization allows for regulation and control of the cannabis market and, ideally, should reduce the burden on the criminal justice system. But it gives the government a lot more control over the industry's development. Decriminalization reduces the severity of penalties for minor cannabis offenses and may reduce the number of arrests, but it does not address public health concerns and does not create room for legal cannabis commerce and, therefore, no industry infrastructure for revenue generation.

Ultimately, legalization should encompass decriminalization as part of its policy framework. Many jurisdictions that have legalized cannabis have also decriminalized its possession and use, recognizing that criminalizing these activities may still have negative consequences and harm individuals and communities. For example, in some US states, while the sale and possession of cannabis may be legal for recreational use, certain amounts of possession outside of regulated channels may still be subject to civil fines rather than criminal charges. The extent to which decriminalization is included in legalization efforts will depend on the specific laws and regulations put in place by lawmakers.

De-scheduling Cannabis

Cannabis was first classified as a Schedule 1 drug under the CSA in 1970 when the CSA was signed into law by President Richard Nixon. Cannabis was placed in Schedule 1 along with other drugs like heroin, which is considered to have a high potential for abuse, no accepted medical use, and a lack of accepted safety for use under medical supervision.

Since then, cannabis has remained a Schedule 1 drug under the CSA despite increasing evidence of its medicinal benefits and changing attitudes toward drug policy. In recent years, there have been efforts by lawmakers and advocates to reclassify or de-schedule cannabis, but these efforts have yet to result in any major changes to federal drug policy.

What does de-scheduling mean? To de-schedule cannabis means to remove it from the list of controlled substances under the federal CSA. Currently, cannabis is invalidly classified as a Schedule I drug under the CSA. I say invalidly because, as stated earlier, to qualify to be on the list, said substances must have a high potential for abuse, no accepted medical use, and a lack of accepted safety for use under medical supervision. There is surmountable scientific evidence to corroborate this notion with respect to cannabis.

Removing cannabis from the list of controlled substances would mean that it is no longer subject to federal criminal penalties or restrictions and would be regulated more like other legal commodities. This would allow for greater flexibility in developing state-based regulatory frameworks for medical or adult use, as well as the further development of a regulated multi-state cannabis industry.

De-scheduling cannabis would also make it easier for researchers to study the potential medical benefits and risks of cannabis use, as it would remove some of the bureaucratic barriers and restrictions currently in place that make it difficult to conduct research on the substance.

It's worth noting that while some lawmakers and advocates have proposed legislation to de-schedule cannabis, this would require significant political will and a major overhaul of federal drug policy as it remains a highly controversial global issue.

Normalization

The normalization movement of the cannabis plant refers to the cultural shift that has occurred over the past several decades, as cannabis has moved from being a stigmatized and taboo substance to one that is increasingly accepted and mainstreamed in society. This shift has been driven by several factors, including changing attitudes toward drug policy, the emergence of the medical cannabis industry, the growing body of research on the potential benefits of cannabis for a range of health conditions, and the remarkable amount of work being done by cannabis advocates around the world.

As part of the normalization movement, there has been a concerted effort to destigmatize and normalize cannabis use, particularly for medical purposes. This has included the development of new products, the vast education of the many available delivery methods for consumption beyond smoking, including edibles, oils, and vaporizers, as well as the marketing of cannabis products using familiar and mainstream imagery, branding, and narrative.

In addition to changes in product design and marketing, the normalization movement has also been characterized by a growing number of high-profile advocates and public figures who openly consume and advocate for the plant, as well as an increasing number of jurisdictions that have legalized cannabis for medical or adult use. All these factors have contributed to a shift in the cultural narrative around cannabis from one of fear and criminality to one of acceptance and normalization.

Social Equity

Social equity in cannabis refers to efforts to address the historical and ongoing injustices and inequities in the criminalization and enforcement of cannabis prohibition and to ensure that the benefits of the legal cannabis industry are accessible to communities that have been disproportionately impacted by the War on Drugs.

The concept of social equity recognizes that many communities, particularly communities of color and low-income communities, have been disproportionately impacted by harsh drug laws and the enforcement of those laws since prohibition started. This has resulted in higher rates of arrest, incarceration, and many negative consequences for these communities and has perpetuated systemic inequality and social injustice.

To address these issues, ideally social equity initiatives aim to make sure that the cannabis industry promotes diversity and inclusion from seed to sale, has programs to provide resources and support for individuals and communities that have been affected by the War on Drugs, and ensure that the benefits of the legal cannabis industry are accessible to a broad range of individuals and communities.

Social equity in cannabis is often associated with racial relations because communities of color have been disproportionately impacted by the War on Drugs and the enforcement of cannabis laws; hence, if you do the math, the beneficiaries of social equity initiatives will be disproportionately Black and Brown folks. The disproportionate impact of drug laws and enforcement on communities of color has been well-documented, with studies showing that Black and Latine individuals are more likely to be arrested, convicted, and incarcerated for drug offenses, including cannabis-related offenses, despite similar rates of drug use among different racial and ethnic groups.

As a result, social equity initiatives in the cannabis industry often focus on providing support and resources for individuals and communities victimized by drug policy. These initiatives may include measures to provide training and support for cannabis entrepreneurs from under-represented communities, create policies that prioritize the hiring of individuals from these communities, and establish equity programs that provide financial and technical assistance to these emerging entrepreneurs.

It's important to note that social equity in cannabis is not solely about race and that individuals from all backgrounds and communities can be and have been impacted by the criminalization of cannabis and the War on Drugs. However, historical evidence shows that Black communities have been the most impacted by cannabis prohibition and the War on Drugs. Thus, Social equity initiatives in the cannabis industry aim to address systemic inequality and promote diversity and inclusion in the regulated industry. Ultimately, the goal is to create a more equitable, inclusive, and just cannabis space.

Pardon vs. Expungement

As I write this book, history unfolds with US President Biden addressing the nation, announcing a monumental act of clemency: mass pardon for individuals convicted of federal cannabis possession. While such bold acts of mass clemency typically entail the release of incarcerated individuals, this one is unique; it won't lead to anyone regaining their freedom. According to a report from the US Sentencing Commission (USSC), there's currently no one in federal custody solely for simple cannabis possession.

Criminal justice professor Barry Latzer, in an opinion piece for the New York Daily News, sheds light on this seemingly paradoxical situation. In 2020, federal courts saw fewer than 800 cannabis possession cases, with approximately half resulting in convictions, often through guilty pleas. Of these convictions, only around 160 translated into prison sentences, with an average term of half a year.

The explanation lies in the fact that federal law enforcement isn't typically engaged in policing activities that lead to drug possession arrests. Except for cases involving interstate travel and specific federal territories such as the US border, drug possession predominantly falls under the jurisdiction of local law enforcement.

This context is essential in understanding why the president encouraged state governors to follow suit by granting mass clemency to individuals incarcerated for state cannabis possession crimes, estimated at around 30,000 people nationwide. It's noteworthy to observe which states align with this approach, as some governors have been proactive in either expunging records or establishing systems for individuals to have their convictions expunged in tandem with state-level cannabis legalization. Predictably, responses from governors, as compiled by news and media organization Marijuana Moment, reveal a partisan divide, with Democrats applauding the move and Republicans voicing criticism.

For eligible individuals, this pardon will restore certain civic rights forfeited due to the felony conviction, such as voting or serving on juries. However, it's crucial to note that pardons do not remove convictions from a person's record; only expungement can achieve that. This distinction marks the difference between the two processes.

Yet, the story doesn't end here. The proposed clemency doesn't encompass individuals found guilty of intent to distribute. Shockingly, there are individuals serving sentences exceeding fifty years for attempting to sell a mere $300 worth of cannabis. This poses a glaring need for reform.

Furthermore, Biden's pardon exclusively applies to citizens and lawful permanent residents, a move that has deeply frustrated immigrant rights advocates. For many years, non-citizens constituted a significant portion of those convicted of simple cannabis possession. In 2014, over 90% of simple possession offenders were detained at the southern border, primarily in Arizona, with about 94% of these arrests involving non-citizens. While these numbers have substantially decreased over the years, it's critical to acknowledge the concerns and complexities surrounding this aspect.

Other pertinent terms:

- 420: A cannabis holiday that occurs on April 20. Also a slang term for cannabis or a cannabis-friendly event, venue, person, or noun/verb in general.
- 710: A cannabis holiday focused on concentrates, observed on July 10. The name comes from flipping the date (710) upside down to resemble the word oil.
- *Adult-use / Recreational*: Adults (21+) who purchase cannabis products at a dispensary and use cannabis products recreationally.
- *Ancillary*: Non-plant-touching businesses in the cannabis industry. These are businesses that service the cannabis operators and other cannabis stakeholders. Examples include tech companies, recruitment businesses, lawyers, Accountants, etc.
- *Broad Spectrum*: This refers to a product that contains all components of the cannabis plant, but the THC has been completely removed.
- *Bud*: Bud is the flower of the cannabis plant that is usually consumed or used to formulate cannabis-derived products. It is also a general slang term for cannabis.
- *Budtender*: A very important retail cannabis employee who assists customers or patients in the shopping process. Usually works at the retail counter and sales floor. A budtender is the main customer point of contact at a retail business.
- *Cannabinoids*: These are the chemical compounds secreted by cannabis flowers that provide relief to an array of symptoms. The most well-known among these include THC and CBD. THC, the cannabinoid prohibitionists love to hate as it is often associated with being responsible for the psychoactive effects that recreational users seek, while CBD, which is federally legal, is mostly associated with therapeutic effects. FYI, there are over 113 known

cannabinoids, and they all work together to provide therapeutic effects.

- *Chemovars:* Also known as chemotypes, refers to the breakdown of a plant species according to its chemical composition. Chemovar classification is pivotal for growers and breeders. Certain chemical characteristics determine, for example, whether a cannabis indica plant has a greater CBD-to-THC ratio or vice versa. It may also determine the presence and bioavailability of certain terpenes.
- *Compliance:* A term used to describe businesses, employees, or actions that are completely legal within the confines of the state's (city or county) cannabis regulations.
- *Concentrates and Extracts:* These terms refer to the product of a process where cannabinoids and terpenes are extracted from the cannabis plant. The primary distinction between a cannabis extract and a cannabis concentrate lies in the extent of their refinement: while an extract has generally been moderately refined to separate out cannabinoids and terpenes, a concentrate has been subjected to a higher degree of refinement and post-processing. Examples include hash, rosin, and waxes.
- *Cultivars or "Strains":* Refer to the myriad types of the plant that have evolved over centuries through a combination of natural selection and deliberate breeding by horticulturists, growers, and scientists. These diverse genetic variations are the culmination of hundreds of years of hybridization and experimentation, shaping the unique characteristics of each strain, from its flavor profile to its psychoactive effects.
- *Dabs/Dabbing:* Dabs or dabbing are cultural words for the consumption of cannabis concentrates.
- *Decarboxylation:* This is a process that involves heating cannabis to activate the compounds within. Raw cannabis

contains THCA and CBDA, which are the acidic forms of THC and CBD. Heating turns these into active forms.

- *Edibles:* These are food products infused with cannabis, often used as an alternative to smoking. They come in many forms, such as brownies, cookies, candies, drinks, and more.
- *Endocannabinoid System (ECS):* This is a complex cell-signaling system in the human body known to play a role in regulating a range of functions and processes, including sleep, mood, appetite, memory, and reproduction and fertility. The ECS interacts with cannabinoids like THC and CBD, which can influence these bodily functions.
- *Entourage Effect:* This refers to the synergistic interaction of the cannabis plant's various compounds that magnify the therapeutic benefits of the plant's individual components — so the medicinal impact of the whole plant is greater than the sum of its parts.
- *Flavonoids:* Naturally occurring compounds responsible for the plant's color, aroma, and flavor. They also contribute to the plant's potential therapeutic effects.
- *Full Spectrum:* Full spectrum means that the product contains all cannabinoids and terpenes found in the cannabis plant.
- *Hash:* Hash, short for hashish, is a concentrated form of cannabis that is made by separating the resin glands (also known as trichomes) from the plant material and compressing them into a solid or semi-solid form. Hash contains a high concentration of cannabinoids, primarily THC (tetrahydrocannabinol) and terpenes, making it more potent than traditional cannabis flowers. Hash is one of the oldest forms of cannabis concentrate, with historical records and uses dating back centuries in various parts of the world, particularly the Middle East and Asia. The methods for producing hash vary, but they generally

involve mechanical or manual separation of trichomes from the cannabis plant followed by a compression process.

- *Hemp:* This is a variety of cannabis plant species that is grown specifically for the industrial uses of its derived products. Its THC content is significantly lower, and it is also the primary source of CBD.
- *Indica, Sativa, and Hybrid:* These are the three main types of cannabis classification at the retail level. Indica strains are believed to be physically sedating and are perfect for relaxation. Sativa strains tend to provide more invigorating, uplifting cerebral effects that pair well with physical activity, social gatherings, and creative projects. Hybrid strains are a blend of both Indica and Sativa strains, offering a balance of effects.
- *Infused:* Refers to the process of incorporating cannabis extracts or concentrates into various types of products such as edibles, beverages, tinctures, topicals, and oils. The infusion allows for cannabinoids (like THC and CBD), terpenes, and other beneficial compounds to be evenly distributed within the product, providing a measured and controlled way to consume cannabis.
- *Medical:* Term for cannabis and cannabis products consumed by medical patients.
- *MIPs:* Acronym for marijuana-infused products. The term refers to any products that are infused with cannabis, such as edibles, tinctures, drinkables, etc.
- *Moonrock:* "Moon Rocks" refers to a specific type of cannabis product designed for a very potent experience. A Moon Rock starts with a whole cannabis bud, which is then coated with a layer of cannabis concentrate like hash oil or butane hash oil (BHO). After applying the concentrate, the bud is rolled in kief, the resinous trichomes that fall off cannabis flowers. The result is a "rock" of cannabis that is

significantly more potent than any individual form of cannabis alone.

- *Plant touching*: Roles in cannabis that handle cannabis directly. Most roles that fall within the cultivation, retail, lab/extraction, and manufacturing roles are considered plant touching.
- *Puff Puff Pass*: An unwritten code of conduct that governs the etiquette of communal smoking sessions. Whether it is friends gathered around a campfire or a circle of acquaintances at a social gathering, this simple mantra dictates the flow of a joint, blunt, spliff, or pre-roll among a group. The idea is straightforward: take two puffs and then pass the smoking implement to the next person in the circle. In some cultures, it is passed to the left. In others, it is passed to the right.
- *Rosin*: Rosin refers to a solventless cannabis concentrate produced using a combination of heat and pressure to extract resin from the plant material. Unlike other concentrates that may use solvents like butane or ethanol in the extraction process, rosin is considered a more natural and pure form of concentrate because it doesn't involve any chemicals.
- *Skunk*: A specific lineage of cannabis strains known for their strong, pungent aroma reminiscent of a skunk's scent. These strains are often high in THC, the psychoactive compound in cannabis, making them popular for both recreational and medical use. The term "Skunk" is sometimes used more broadly to describe any high-THC cannabis with a similarly strong smell, although this usage is not technically accurate.
- *Terpenes*: These are the fragrant oils that give cannabis its aromatic diversity. They're secreted in the same glands that produce cannabinoids. Terpenes also play a key role in differentiating the effects of various cannabis strains.

- *Tincture:* A cannabis extract produced by immersing the plant in substances like alcohol, glycerin, or oil. This process yields liquid rich in cannabinoids, terpenes, and flavonoids, which can be ingested in many ways, such as sublingually or orally.
- *Topical:* A transdermal way to use cannabis. Topicals serve as lubricants that go beyond just the skin's surface layer. Cannabis topicals function by directly entering the bloodstream through the skin (ex., salves, balms, creams).
- *Trichomes:* "Fine outgrowths or appendages on plants, algae, lichens, and certain protists." In cannabis, these are where the production of the hundreds of known cannabinoids, terpenes, and flavonoids that make the strains we love potent, unique, and effective.
- *Wake and Bake:* The act of smoking cannabis shortly after waking up in the morning. This morning ritual is a cherished routine for many cannabis enthusiasts.
- *Wax:* A dense, shelf-stable, and highly potent extraction of cannabinoids such as THC and CBD, as well as flavorful compounds such as terpenes and flavonoids.

Canna-Math

Cannabis measurements are a part of the cannabis culture. A basic understanding of cannabis math comes in handy at the counter when shopping for it, when carrying legal amounts in public, or when testing cannabis products in a lab. At a dispensary, for instance, cannabis is available in various measurements such as grams, eighths, half-ounces, and ounces. Each form—whether it's flower, pre-rolled joints, vapes, or concentrates—has its unique measurement standards, making it crucial to grasp these metrics to ensure informed decision-making with respect to consumption, storing or purchasing.

Cannabis Weight Breakdown:

- *Gram:* Typically, the smallest quantity of cannabis flower you can buy at a dispensary is one gram. This amount is usually sufficient for rolling one to two joints.
- *Eighth:* An eighth of cannabis, commonly referred to simply as an eighth, measures 3.5 grams. This term originates from its proportionate relation to an ounce; specifically, it is one-eighth of an ounce. Hence, eight eighths make up one full ounce.
- *Quarter:* A quarter, representing a quarter of an ounce, equates to seven grams. It's sometimes abbreviated to 'Q' in slang terminology.
- *Half Ounce:* A half ounce, or 'half-O,' amounts to 14 grams. This terminology simplifies the reference to half of a full ounce.
- *Ounce:* An ounce of cannabis, which is about 28.5 grams, is often the maximum quantity an individual can legally possess at one time in various states, like California. This limit includes an allowance to carry an additional 8 grams of cannabis concentrate. The ounce serves as a fundamental unit in cannabis transactions globally.
- *Pound:* One pound of cannabis equals 16 ounces or approximately 448 grams. In slang, a pound is often referred to as a "pack" or "elbow."

Chapter 10
The Culture is Not for Sale

Cannabis culture has fascinated me for years, resonating deeply with my own experiences and observations. As I perceive it, it is a complex ecosystem of social attitudes, historical legacies, and ever-changing practices centered around this remarkable plant. The culture transcends its ancient origins, when it was revered for its medicinal and spiritual properties, to carve a niche in modern society where it's far more than just a "substance'—it's a way of life.

We've discussed how cannabis has been around for millennia, its therapeutic roots tracing back to ancient China around 2700 BC. From there, it traveled the globe, embedding itself in diverse customs and traditions, from textile manufacturing to religious rites. So, when some people imagine that cannabis culture was born in the 1960s alongside the American counterculture movement, they're only seeing a fraction of the whole picture. While the '60s and '70s were transformative—casting cannabis as a symbol of rebellion, communal living, and personal freedom—it was also the period when the "War on Drugs" dramatically escalated the stakes, particularly in the US, criminalizing cannabis use and deepening the cultural divide.

Even when faced with these draconian policies, cannabis culture found ways to blossom. It continued to influence popular culture, epitomized by icons like Bob Marley and the rise of 420 as a code term that evolved into a symbol of unity and resistance. The latter part of the twentieth century and the early years of the twenty-first have seen a seismic shift in attitudes. Medical cannabis initiatives and legalization campaigns across the globe have prompted a reassessment, and the stigma that once loomed over cannabis has started to fade.

Today, the face of cannabis culture is a multifaceted one. It's no longer confined to the act of smoking; it's a lifestyle that integrates the plant in manifold ways. From cannabis-infused cuisine and fashion lines celebrating the plant to an array of health and wellness products centered around its medicinal properties, the cultural impact is sprawling. Then there's the burgeoning legal industry, offering not just a plethora of products but also opportunities for entrepreneurship and job creation.

At its core, cannabis culture is a social justice movement. The destructive effects of the War on Drugs, particularly its disproportionate impact on BIPOC communities, cannot be overstated. Activists today are fighting not just for the plant's legalization but for equitable opportunities within the cannabis industry and the expungement of past nonviolent cannabis-related offenses.

The culture's diversity reflects its participants: professionals, parents, seniors, athletes, and individuals from all cultural and social strata, even animals. Far from the cliché of the lazy stoner, the community is an amalgamation of innovation, creativity, and a quest for freedom—personal and social in nature. Despite the lingering legal battles and societal misconceptions, one thing is for sure: the culture is here to stay.

At its most basic, cannabis culture is about a plant that has the power to bring people together. It's a common thread that weaves through various aspects of life, from social relaxation and medical relief to activism and advocacy. As we venture into an era where cannabis gains more widespread acceptance, its cultural influence is poised to expand in ways we can only begin to imagine. In that sense, it's not just a culture but a testament to human ingenuity, resilience, natural therapy, and the perpetual quest for a more tolerant and inclusive society.

Vipers and the Gage: A Revolutionary Act

Early beginnings in the good ol' US of A...Many people associate jazz with cannabis, but most don't know the "stoner" culture began with jazz and blues artists. Their term for a cannabis smoker was "Viper." Let's talk about it!

In the chronicles of American culture, few relationships are as fascinating as the symbiotic one between jazz and cannabis. Many of us know that jazz and "reefer" go hand-in-hand, but few realize that this alliance practically inaugurated what we call "stoner culture" today. Back then, the individuals who openly appreciated the cannabis smoking experience were jazz musicians, and they called themselves "Vipers."

It's nearly impossible to talk about the evolution of jazz without recognizing its roots in Black communities. This powerful art form, founded by Black musicians, provided fertile ground for the intimate relationship between jazz and cannabis. For musicians like Louis Armstrong, Lester Young, and Billie Holiday, cannabis wasn't just a recreational escape; it was a catalyst for creativity, a muse for musical composition, and a magical ingredient in their spellbinding performances.

The term "Viper" came into play during the 1920s and 1930s, an era where cannabis use was stigmatized and prohibited. In this volatile landscape, jazz musicians—defiant and irrepressible—found solace and inspiration in cannabis. They had a myriad of code names for it—Mary Jane, tea, grass, gage—each one a discreet nod to the noteworthy plant. These Vipers didn't just use cannabis; they celebrated it—incorporating their love for it into their lyrics and boldly renaming strains to suit their artistic whims.

Louis Armstrong, a jazz legend and quintessential Viper, had a particularly intimate relationship with cannabis. Armstrong asserted that "it enhanced his creativity, improved his performance, and even increased his appreciation of music." Moreover, Armstrong found in cannabis an emotional sanctuary, a refuge from the racial injustices of the time. When he smoked with a fellow Viper, he said, they could *"forget all the bad things that happen to a negro,"* highlighting the plant's role as a coping mechanism amid racial tensions experienced at the time.

It's this transformative era that inspired the third collection of my advocacy lifestyle brand, Boycott Shitty Weed (BSW Nation). The VIPERS collection serves as an homage to these fearless jazz artists who, in a climate of stigma and criminalization, lifted their joints high. Through the Vipers campaign, we aim to ignite a cultural dialogue, challenging long-standing stigmas and acknowledging the substantial role that cannabis played in this iconic era of American music and social history.

As we extend our advocacy into the digital frontier, BSW Nation has even entered the metaverse, creating a safe space for cannabis enthusiasts of all types—advocates, connoisseurs, canna-preneurs, and the canna-curious. Within this digital realm, we host events, showcase a Viper gallery, and create social clubs to keep the conversation going, applying a modern twist to a profoundly influential era.

The Vipers of the past were unapologetic in their celebration of cannabis and its artistic influence. In capturing this spirit, we hope to be just as fearless in confronting the stigmas that have long plagued this extraordinary plant. The tide of Vipers was unstoppable back then; it remains so today, its influence rippling through the cannabis and jazz communities alike.

Reefer Madness

Reefer Madness is a term that refers to the propaganda campaign in the 1930s that demonized cannabis use and spread false information about its effects on individuals and society. The campaign depicted cannabis as a dangerous drug that could lead to insanity, violence, and moral decay.

The campaign was primarily led by government officials and media outlets, and it was used to justify the prohibition of cannabis. The message of Reefer Madness was that cannabis consumption was not only harmful to the individual but also a threat to society as a whole.

The implications of Reefer Madness were far-reaching. It created a stigma around cannabis consumption that persists to this day. The propaganda campaign led to the criminalization of cannabis, and it was used to justify the War on Drugs, which, by now, we all know, disproportionately affected communities of color.

The misinformation spread by Reefer Madness also led to a lack of research on the potential benefits of the cannabis plant, as its federal status prevents funding for much-needed scientific studies. As we have discussed throughout the book, it wasn't until the twenty-first century that attitudes toward cannabis began to change due to the many personal experiences and the availability of research conducted into its potential benefits in several countries.

Flower Children and Smoke Rings: Hippies and the Counterculture Movement

In the United States, the connection between cannabis and the hippie movement of the 1960s and 1970s holds a critical place in the history of cannabis culture. It was a period when cannabis gained immense popularity among the youth, especially those aligned with the counterculture movement.

The hippies embraced cannabis to challenge mainstream cultural norms and advocate for a more inclusive and peaceful society. For them, using cannabis was more than mere recreation—it was a cultural act, serving as a gateway to deeper connections with nature and fellow human beings. Of course, cannabis wasn't the only substance they utilized for these purposes. ;)

Prominent figures within the counterculture movement played

vital roles in influencing public perception of cannabis. Some key advocates include:

- *Allen Ginsberg:* A leading voice of the Beat Generation, Ginsberg not only advocated for cannabis but took substantial actions, such as co-founding the pro-legalization group LeMar (Legalize Marijuana) and organizing the first medical marijuana conference in 1964.
- *Timothy Leary:* More famous for his promotion of psychedelics like LSD, Leary was also a crucial advocate for cannabis. His legal battle against his own arrest for marijuana possession led to the landmark Supreme Court case Leary v. United States, which found the Marihuana Tax Act of 1937 unconstitutional.
- *Tom Forçade:* The man behind High Times magazine, founded in 1974, Forçade was instrumental in fostering cannabis culture. The magazine not only called for marijuana legalization but served as a hub for discussing cultivation techniques, reviewing strains, and amplifying the cannabis movement's cultural and political ethos (more about High Times as you read along).
- *Peter Tosh:* A prominent musician and an integral part of the reggae movement, Tosh was a fierce advocate for the legalization of marijuana, often emphasizing its spiritual and medicinal importance. His famous song "Legalize It" became an anthem for cannabis advocacy and remains influential to this day.
- *The San Francisco Diggers:* Active in the late 1960s, this group advocated for a free society that endorsed the open use of the plant. They organized free events and "happenings" where cannabis was shared, adding a communal aspect to its consumption.

These individuals, along with the handful mentioned in chapter 4 and many more, each in their unique way, helped reshape public opinion about cannabis during this era. As these decades developed, the opposition also developed narratives to reinforce the stigma, causing the "stoner" stereotype to emerge, painting cannabis users as lazy and detached from societal responsibilities. While this stereotype cemented the countercultural status of cannabis, it also "complicated" its image (for lack of a better term).

Today, although the plant's association with hippie culture has significantly diminished, cannabis consumption has become increasingly mainstream and endorsed by various communities and subcultures. Nevertheless, the hippie era's legacy still echoes in the modern cultural landscape surrounding cannabis.

In contemporary society, cannabis has transcended its countercultural roots to represent a broad spectrum of social norms. It's now often linked with relaxation, therapeutic relief, creativity, and a strong sense of community. This evolution has greatly impacted the development of the legal cannabis industry, with cannabis-centric events like festivals, concerts, and trade shows growing in popularity, fostering a sense of community and unity among consumers and advocates alike.

Amsterdam: The First Cannabis Oasis

Since the Netherlands decriminalized cannabis in 1976, it's been a bucket-list destination for cannabis enthusiasts. Amsterdam often conjures images of bustling "coffee shops" where cannabis is openly consumed, leading many to mistakenly think the plant is legal in the Netherlands. The reality is more nuanced; cannabis isn't actually legal but rather decriminalized for personal use. Dutch law still technically prohibits the recreational use, possession, and trade of drugs listed under the Opium Law, which includes cannabis. However, since the late twentieth century, the government has adopted a policy of toleration, particularly for personal use and possession of small amounts, effectively turning a blind eye to these activities under certain circumstances. This pragmatic stance stems from the acknowledgment that striving for a completely drug-free society is both unrealistic and impractical. Instead, the focus is on harm reduction, aiming to minimize the adverse effects of recreational drug use.

In a bid to combat the negative aspects of cannabis tourism, Amsterdam's Mayor has proposed far-reaching regulations that could have a ripple effect on the global cannabis tourism industry, currently estimated to be worth $17 billion annually. New policies in Amsterdam's central tourist area include limiting alcohol sales, enforcing earlier bar closures, and issuing €100 ($107) fines for public cannabis consumption. The mayor characterizes cannabis tourism as a source of crime and public disorder, even suggesting the controversial step of prohibiting foreigners from accessing the city's famed cannabis cafés.

With cannabis regulations loosening worldwide in places like Thailand, South Africa, Uruguay, Jamaica, Malta, Mexico, Canada, and the United States, the tourism landscape could be primed for major changes as travelers may seek alternative destinations that offer less stringent cannabis-related laws.

The 420 Code

Cannabis culture is also closely tied to the concept of "420," which has become a shorthand for cannabis culture and pretty much cannabis-anything. The origins of the term are somewhat murky, but it is believed to have originated in the 1970s in California as a code among high school students for cannabis use. Over time, the term "four-twenty" (420) became associated with cannabis culture more broadly and came to represent a shared identity and sense of community among cannabis consumers and advocates. The Grateful Dead, a legendary American rock band closely associated with the counterculture and the psychedelic music scene of the 1960s, also played a role in popularizing "420" as a code for cannabis. The band and their fans, known as Deadheads, are often credited with helping spread its use.

The term has been embraced by a wide range of subcultures, and has been featured in music, film, media, and other forms of popular culture. Today, 420 is celebrated annually on April 20, with cannabis-related events, festivals, concerts, and other gatherings taking place around the world.

A few years ago a good friend by the name of Shagwhelin Bullock (a.k.a. Shaggy) introduced me to *The 420 Code: A Guide to the "High Life" and Cannabis Culture*. The author remains anonymous, but he took the time to materialize the 420 philosophy, encompassing four "virtues" and twenty "rules of thumb." These are a set of principles and guidelines for those who embrace cannabis as part of their lifestyle. The fact that it has been widely read and even turned into a pocketbook, with multiple printings, shows that it has resonated with many people in the cannabis community.

Furthermore, the full text is available for free at www.the420 code.com. The author stays true to the spirit of sharing knowledge and promoting a sense of community often associated with cannabis culture. Those who appreciate creative ways to express the cannabis culture and philosophy surrounding cannabis might find The 420 Code guide meaningful and valuable.

Ultimately, the culture of cannabis is a rich and diverse phenomenon that reflects the many ways in which cannabis has been embraced by different communities throughout history. The aforementioned is why I personally love the culture so much and the reason why I firmly believe that as cannabis continues to become accepted and more mainstream, the culture will continue to evolve and adapt to changing social and cultural norms.

Sinsemilla

Sinsemilla, often spelled in varying ways like sensimilla or sinse, refers to unfertilized female cannabis plants, which leads to a boost in the plant's cannabinoid and terpene profiles. This cultivation method originally gained traction in Sinaloa, Mexico, in the '70s, thanks to drug kingpin Rafael Caro Quintero, who determined that the key to this process is to identify and remove male plants early to prevent them from pollinating the females. The purpose is to produce seedless bud that is more pleasurable for recreational consumption and to divert the plant's energy from producing seeds to producing higher levels of cannabinoids such as THC.

This technique exploded in popularity in the US, elevating the THC content in cannabis significantly. A 1980 study showed that while street cannabis had an average THC content of 1.8%, sinsemilla strains clocked in at 6%. Sinsemilla is a cultivation technique. Many do confuse it as a "strain" or cultivar. Also, don't confuse it with "skunk," which refers to specific high-THC strains.

While the term "sinsemilla" may sound a bit dated today, especially with the advent of feminized seeds in the '90s, its impact on cannabis cultivation is undeniable. These feminized seeds are essentially engineered to always produce female plants, making the separation of male plants almost a thing of the past.

Cornerstones of Cannabis Culture

While the cultural acceptance of cannabis has roots in various subcultures, from the Vipers of the Jazz Age to the hippies of the counterculture era, the work of advocacy organizations cannot be overlooked in shaping the contemporary landscape of cannabis in America. These organizations have been the backbone of a movement that sought to decriminalize, legalize, and normalize cannabis use for medical and adult-use purposes. More than just platforms for legal reform, they've also been critical in shifting public perception and fostering a more accepting and informed culture around the plant.

Whether working through grassroots campaigns, educational outreach, or legislative lobbying, these organizations have taken on the establishment at every level. They've made strides in overturning long-standing stigmas, in part by working to correct misinformation and highlight the medicinal and economic benefits of the plant, as well as the detriment set forth by prohibition. Their role has been multifaceted, working not just to impact legal change but also to create a space where activists could coordinate, share information, and even celebrate the rich history and potential future of a world where cannabis is no longer stigmatized.

In the following paragraphs, we will discuss the stories of some of these pioneering organizations. Each one has its own unique approach and focus—some championing the medicinal aspects of cannabis, others tackling the social justice implications of its criminalization, and others emphasizing its cultural and economic importance. But what they all share is a commitment to bringing cannabis out of the shadows and into the mainstream discourse, forever altering the trajectory of the history of the plant in society.

NORML

The first cannabis advocacy organization to be established in the United States was the NORML. NORML was founded in 1970 by attorney Keith Stroup. The organization was created to advocate for the legalization of cannabis in America.

At the time of its founding, NORML was one of the few organizations working to promote cannabis policy reform. It played a crucial role in shaping the cultural and legal landscape surrounding cannabis use back then. In the years since its founding, NORML has grown to become one of the most well-known and influential cannabis advocacy organizations in the world and continues to play a significant role in many state-level legalization efforts. NORML remains a voice in the legalization movement and has played a significant role in advancing medical cannabis policy and advocacy in the US.

The Cannabis Action Network (CAN)

The Cannabis Action Network (CAN) was a non-profit organization that advocated for the legalization of cannabis and the end of the War on Drugs. The organization was founded in 1992 in Washington, DC, by Richard Cowan, a former director of NORML.

CAN worked to promote education and awareness about cannabis and advocated for policies that prioritize public health and safety. The organization supported harm reduction strategies, such as drug education and access to treatment, and worked to reduce the negative consequences of drug prohibition.

One of the primary goals of CAN was to empower individuals and communities to become active participants in the cannabis legalization movement. CAN played a role in many state-level cannabis legalization efforts and was involved in the development of several state-level ballot initiatives. The organization also worked to promote federal and state specific policy reform.

While CAN is no longer active, its work has had a positive impact on the cannabis legalization movement in America. The organization's advocacy helped to shape the cultural and political landscape surrounding cannabis use and cannabis policy and contributed to the growing momentum for cannabis policy reform in the 1990s.

The Marijuana Policy Project (MPP)

The Marijuana Policy Project (MPP) is a non-profit organization that advocates for the legalization and regulation of cannabis in the US. The organization was founded in 1995 by Rob Kampia, Chuck Thomas, and Mike Kirshner. The organization has played a significant role in many state-level cannabis legalization efforts.

MPP works to promote cannabis policy reform at the state and federal levels and advocates for policies that prioritize public health and safety. The organization promotes harm reduction strategies, such as access to treatment and education, and works to reduce the negative consequences of cannabis prohibition.

One of the primary goals of MPP is to empower individuals and communities. The organization provides resources and training for individuals who are interested in getting involved in cannabis policy advocacy and offers a platform for individuals and organizations to share their experiences and perspectives on policy reform. The organization has also been a vocal advocate for the reform of federal cannabis policy and has worked to promote policies that prioritize public health and safety. The organization's work has helped to shape the cultural and political landscape surrounding the cannabis plant.

Students for Sensible Drug Policy (SSDP)

Students for Sensible Drug Policy (SSDP) has been an instrumental force in driving change within the realm of drug policy in the United States. Founded in 1998, this non-profit organization was conceived by a collective of concerned college students. They aimed to tackle the detrimental effects of drug prohibition on both individual lives and broader communities.

With a focus on youth engagement, SSDP mobilizes students and young adults to advocate for more sensible and humane policies. Their initiatives underscore harm reduction approaches, such as comprehensive drug abuse education and increased access to treatment programs.

SSDP's commitment to empowering the youth is evident in its comprehensive range of training programs and resources tailored specifically for young activists. This approach not only equips them with the tools necessary to impact change but also fosters a sense of community by providing platforms for like-minded individuals to connect and share experiences.

In the arena of cannabis legalization, SSDP has been a formidable player. The organization has contributed substantially to state-level legalization efforts and has been an influential voice in shaping public opinion. Moreover, their advocacy extends beyond cannabis to include policy reform for other controlled substances, particularly in the realms of opioid use and overdose prevention.

As a grassroots entity, the influence of SSDP reaches far and wide. Its dedication to drug policy reform has not only instigated change at the legislative level but also significantly impacted the cultural narrative surrounding drug abuse in America. Through its tireless efforts, SSDP has undeniably contributed to creating a more compassionate and rational framework for drug abuse policy in the United States.

The International Association for Cannabinoid Medicines (IACM)

The International Association for Cannabinoid Medicines (IACM) stands as a pivotal organization in the field of medical cannabis advocacy. Founded in 2000 by Dr. Franjo Grotenhermen, a distinguished German physician and cannabis researcher, the IACM has been relentlessly championing the cause of medical cannabis access and research on an international level.

Focused on the intersection of science, medicine, and policy, the IACM aims to be a conduit for evidence-based standards concerning the therapeutic use of cannabis and cannabinoids. By doing so, the organization endeavors to ensure that medical cannabis is both safely administered and legally accessible to patients in need.

A cornerstone of IACM's mission is to catalyze research exploring the medical applications of cannabis. Through its efforts, the organization aims to provide a robust scientific foundation that can guide the development of innovative treatments and therapies centered around cannabinoids. Beyond research, IACM takes an active role in educating healthcare professionals. Through its various programs and initiatives, it seeks to arm clinicians with the knowledge and resources needed to safely and effectively integrate cannabis-based treatments into their practices.

As part of its educational and informational initiatives, IACM publishes the Journal of Cannabis and Cannabinoid Research. This quarterly journal serves as a scholarly platform where researchers and healthcare professionals can disseminate their findings, advancing the collective understanding of cannabis as medicine. Further adding to the organization's impact is its annual Cannabinoid Conference, a global gathering that unites researchers, clinicians, and policymakers to discuss the latest breakthroughs and policy shifts in the realm of medical cannabis.

With its multi-pronged approach to research promotion, education, and policy advocacy, the IACM has emerged as a significant influencer in shaping the global narrative on medical cannabis. In fact, the organization has not only pushed the boundaries of cannabis science but also laid the groundwork for compassionate and evidence-based healthcare policies involving cannabis and cannabinoids.

Americans for Safe Access (ASA)

Americans for Safe Access serves as a critical advocacy and support group in the realm of medical cannabis. Established in 2002, the non-profit organization has continually been a vanguard in the medical cannabis landscape, focusing its efforts on influencing policy, fostering research, educating various stakeholders, and offering much-needed legal aid.

At the heart of ASA's mission is its tireless advocacy work. The organization maintains a robust presence at federal, state, and local levels, pushing for legislation and regulations that are designed to ensure both safe and legal access to medical cannabis. By engaging directly with lawmakers and decision-makers, ASA works to illuminate the potential medical benefits of cannabis and actively counters prevailing myths and disinformation.

Navigating the labyrinthine legal structures surrounding medical cannabis can be a daunting task for patients, caregivers, and even healthcare providers. ASA has programs that offer comprehensive legal guidance, from clarifying state-specific regulations to federal laws. Moreover, they offer essential resources and support for those entangled in legal complications stemming from their medical cannabis use.

In addition to policy reform, ASA places a significant emphasis on research, aiming to cultivate a body of evidence that can substantiate the medical efficacy of cannabis. This focus entails pushing for increased federal and state funding for medical cannabis research, as well as advocating for the removal of bureaucratic hurdles that hinder comprehensive scientific exploration.

Beyond legalities and research, ASA's holistic approach encompasses empowering patients and patient advocates. By offering educational resources, guidance, and opportunities for community engagement, ASA paves ways for the safe access of medical cannabis and serves as informed contributors to the broader conversation on the plant's role in healthcare.

With its multi-faceted approach, Americans for Safe Access has been instrumental in shifting the medical cannabis paradigm, achieving notable success in facilitating safe and legal access for patients. Its sustained efforts have been pivotal in shaping the medical cannabis landscape in our nation, making it an indispensable player in the broader medical cannabis movement.

Terrie Best, the chair of San Diego's Chapter of ASA and ASA's 2015 Activist of the Year, stands as a powerful example of advocacy driven by empathy and a natural hunger for social justice. Her journey into activism was spurred by a deep-rooted compassion for the victims of the drug war, fueling consistent and high-impact work over the years.

Terrie's revolutionary use of grassroots reporting during the trials of medical cannabis patients like Eugene Davidovich and Jovan Jackson became a resource of information for the community. Her efforts laid the groundwork for a more organized approach to cannabis advocacy in our hometown, San Diego, CA.

Terrie's advocacy wasn't inspired by distant observation but by intimate encounters with patients and vulnerable communities. Social justice is at the core of her activism. Despite medical cannabis being legalized in California in 1996, Terrie saw firsthand how the benefits were not being shared equitably across all communities. She found that non-white patients were more likely to plead guilty due to a lack of community and legal support, prompting her to address this inequity with the full force of her advocacy efforts.

Through her leadership role at San Diego ASA, she's facilitated access to crucial legal resources and arranged for expert testimony in court trials. These efforts have led to several acquittals and made her a key resource for attorneys in the area. Terrie believes in maintaining constant pressure on public officials, holding them accountable for their actions through social media and direct confrontations. Whether picketing DEA raids or engaging politicians online, at City Hall, or at protests, she's shown that continuous, strategic pressure can create real change.

Terrie Best's activism goes beyond individual endeavor; it serves as a shining example of the substantial impact a committed person can have on both the community and the larger system. As she frames it, "We have come a long way in San Diego," and her influence and the work of ASA have directly influenced that change in a positive way. With the right mix of passion, resources, and persistence, Terrie shows that it's entirely possible to change the narrative surrounding medical cannabis and social equity.

I'm honored to partner with Terrie Best and MeGain McCall on San Diego's ASA's newest initiative, the Roll Up for Equity campaign and documentary film. This campaign builds on the tradition of community-driven advocacy by providing lawmakers with concrete data about San Diego residents' views on medical cannabis and social equity in cannabis.

In 2022, the city of San Diego initiated the process to include social equity into its cannabis ordinance, a move that was met with resistance from several established operators who saw it as increased competition to their established businesses. They were especially concerned about the perceived advantage granted to potential licensees under the social equity framework. Observing this resistance, Terrie mobilized San Diego ASA, giving rise to the Roll Up for Equity campaign. Its primary goal: to ensure fairness and equity within San Diego's regulated cannabis industry. As of September 8, 2023, the campaign remains active, and San Diego has yet to fully incorporate an equity program in its cannabis ordinance.

Consequently, groups from San Diego's chapter of Americans for Safe Access, the San Diego Blue Dream Democratic Club, and San

Diego NORML have been actively gathering feedback through the campaign's signature postcards. These cards capture voter status and provide sections to denote veteran or senior status. Moreover, they present specific questions, helping to ascertain public sentiment on topics like local cannabis access, consumption lounges, and the need for social equity in the local cannabis sector.

The intention behind the Roll Up for Equity campaign is not just to inform but to empower. As lawmakers deliberate on creating a social equity ordinance and revising land use codes, they will now have a tangible resource that reflects the voice of the community. The postcards serve as more than just a data collection tool; they are a representation of the collective desire for change and equity in San Diego's cannabis landscape.

We're fully committed to this cause and will continue our work until the city's legal cannabis industry reflects the diversity and needs of all its residents. By creating a channel through which everyday people can directly influence policy, we're one step closer to achieving an equitable and accessible medical cannabis industry in San Diego.

The work of Americans for Safe Access and dedicated activists like Terrie Best underscores the transformative power of community advocacy in shaping more compassionate and sensible policies. Through initiatives like the Roll Up for Equity campaign, ASA and its partners are going beyond traditional advocacy. They are democratizing the legislative process, giving voice to those who have been marginalized, and providing lawmakers with the tools they need to enact meaningful change. This #synergy of grassroots activism and data-driven strategy exemplifies the next chapter in medical cannabis advocacy, a chapter focused on access, equity, justice, community, and empowerment.

Blooming Forward

It's crucial to underscore the central principles of compassion, education, advocacy, and community that form the core of the cannabis culture. These are not merely abstract ideas; they embody the essence of what it means to be a part of this green renaissance. Businesses that sidestep these core principles often face many challenges as they lose touch with the very culture they aim to serve.

The cannabis industry is inextricably linked to the culture from which it arose. Those who ignore this truth risk being completely disconnected from the lifeblood of the industry–its people. For that reason, the importance of understanding and honoring the roots and evolution of cannabis culture cannot be overstated, especially for those looking to be a part of it. The culture of cannabis forms the cornerstone for shaping not just a strategic approach but also the vision, mission, and values of all entities operating within this space.

While doing the research for this book, I confirmed what I had been experiencing since I began my journey in cannabis: that the culture of cannabis isn't just an incidental attribute; it's the very soul of this thriving industry. As a stakeholder in this space, recognizing and respecting this isn't optional. In fact, this notion is fundamental to the survival and success of any cannabis centric enterprise, including the governmental kinds. As we navigate the complexities of this green landscape, we must remember that, at its core, cannabis is more than a commodity—it's a community. It's a cause. And most importantly, it's a culture. And no matter how commercially successful it becomes: <u>the culture is not for sale.</u>

As we conclude this chapter, let's take away the understanding that the cannabis industry, with its profound cultural ties, calls for an approach that extends beyond mere commerce. It calls for an approach that recognizes and values the culture that has brought us to this pivotal point in history. We must carry this understanding forward, ensuring that as the cannabis industry continues to bloom, it remains firmly rooted in the rich cultural soil from which it sprung.

Chapter 11
The New Normal

The metamorphosis of cannabis from a marginal, stigmatized substance to a central element in contemporary mainstream culture has been nothing short of revolutionary. Decades of activism, research, and policy reform have cleared a path for this transformation. In many aspects, what we're witnessing today is a cultural shift of seismic proportions. It's no longer just about arguing for decriminalization or the medical benefits of cannabis. The discourse has matured; it now includes nuanced conversations about equity, innovation, justice, the right to do business fairly, and the plant's multidimensional impact on various aspects of society.

The plant's ubiquity in today's culture isn't an isolated phenomenon; it is the sum of a multitude of forces converging at once. Lawmakers are increasingly open to reform as legal cannabis markets demonstrate their potential and the plant's medicinal value continues to surge. The public's perception of cannabis has undergone a radical change, supported by empirical research, and the normalization of cannabis use in media and popular narratives. Even the medical community, traditionally a cautious stakeholder, has started to embrace the therapeutic potentials of cannabinoids, thereby, influencing the health and wellness industry.

But cannabis's influence isn't limited to legal, recreational, and medical realms, it has deeply permeated the arts and creative fields. Writers, musicians, filmmakers, and artists have found both inspiration and refuge in cannabis, channeling their experiences into works that defy conventional boundaries and challenge societal norms. From iconic music albums and Oscar-nominated films to groundbreaking artworks and fashion trends, cannabis has been a muse, a catalyst, and sometimes a co-conspirator in the creative process.

The technological world hasn't been immune to this wave either. Innovations in cultivation, extraction, and distribution are not just scientific endeavors but also a form of creative expression. Even in sectors like architecture and urban planning, the influence of cannabis is palpable, as designers consider sustainable hemp-based materials and integrate cannabis facilities into community spaces.

Perhaps most intriguingly, cannabis has become a prism through which complex spiritual and existential questions are explored. The age-old association of cannabis with spiritual rituals and shamanistic practices is being reexamined in contemporary contexts, contributing to evolving perspectives on spirituality, consciousness, and the human experience.

It is evident that cannabis's impact on mainstream culture is a testament to its multifaceted nature. One of the things that fascinates me about cannabis is how it has not just entered the mainstream but has also fundamentally altered its currents. From stigmatized to celebrated, from marginal to central, the story of cannabis is a mirror to the complexities and contradictions of society itself, inviting us to question, explore, and, ultimately, to embrace a new normal.

The hard work of activists, advocates, and supporters of all walks of life, has caused attitudes toward cannabis to shift significantly in the last couple of decades. The counterculture movement of the late mid-1900s introduced cannabis to a wider audience, presenting it as a symbol of rebellion, freedom, and alternative lifestyle. As the decades passed, this representation has gradually transitioned into mainstream acceptance, driven by an increasingly refined understanding of the plant.

From a legal perspective, the end of the twentieth century and the early twenty-first century marked a significant shift in cannabis policies worldwide. A handful of countries and states have moved toward decriminalizing or legalizing cannabis, particularly for medicinal use. This change in legal status has helped remove some of the stigma associated with cannabis, leading to more open discussions about its use and benefits.

Moreover, scientific research has played a critical role in reshaping public perception of cannabis. Studies highlighting the potential therapeutic applications of cannabinoids, such as CBD, THC, CBN, CBG and others, have contributed to an increased acceptance of cannabis as a legitimate medicinal substance. This has bolstered support for cannabis within the public discourse.

Additionally, the internet and social media have been influential in fostering a more positive and open dialogue around cannabis. Online platforms have made it easier to disseminate information, share personal experiences, and organize advocacy efforts. This has allowed for a more informed discussion debunking common myths and challenging persistent stereotypes.

The commercial potential of cannabis has also been a significant factor in its rising cultural influence. The burgeoning legal cannabis industry, spanning from cultivation and retail to ancillary services and technology, has demonstrated the economic benefits of legalization even with all the hurdles, red tape, over regulation and over taxation. This has not only furthered the argument for legalization but has also helped in the fight for the normalization of cannabis as an everyday consumer product.

Media and Entertainment

In the realm of entertainment, the portrayal of cannabis has shifted dramatically over the years. It's transformed from a rebellious, criminal element to a mainstream topic discussed openly. In the early days, cannabis was mostly presented through stoner comedies such as Cheech and Chong's *Up in Smoke* and *Fast Times at Ridgemont High* which showed cannabis usage as a comedic element intertwined with rebellion against the norm. We can't deny that there is truth behind these narratives as every now and then one comes across a cultivar that gives you the giggles (for me is the White Buffalo strain). But cannabis also helps people to relax, to be creative, to be energetic. Not to mention, smoking is not the only way to consume it.

Most recently, television series and films have started to explore complex narratives around cannabis consumers. The groundbreaking scripted series "Weeds," for instance, showcased a suburban widow who turns to selling marijuana to support her family, challenging the stereotype of typical cannabis users and dealers. More recent series, such as "Disjointed" (2017–2018), portray cannabis dispensaries as normal businesses. Several reality TV shows, including "Weed Country" and "Growing Belushi," focus on cannabis cultivation.

Films like "How High" (2001) and others of its kind have played a significant role in showcasing cannabis use within mainstream culture. These films, often comedic in nature, have brought cannabis use into the public consciousness, moving it away from the shadows and sparking discussions about its societal implications. It was one of the earliest films to present cannabis in a casual, everyday context, an approach that has become increasingly prevalent in more recent years.

Other films that fit into this category include classics like *The Big Lebowski*, as well as more recent films like *Pineapple Express* and *Harold & Kumar Go to White Castle*. These movies feature a range of characters and scenarios, but they all share a common thread: cannabis use is portrayed as a normal part of the characters' lives, not an aberration.

This normalization in popular culture reflects and contributes to the shifting perceptions of cannabis in society at large. As cannabis has become more accepted and less stigmatized, its portrayal in film and television has obviously evolved. It's no longer used solely as a punchline; instead, it's presented as a choice of lifestyle. This bold presentation does not go by without controversy. Critics argue that they may downplay the potential negative consequences of cannabis use and promote its recreational use, especially among impressionable younger audiences. Supporters, on the other hand, contend that these films reflect changing societal attitudes and help destigmatize a substance that has been unfairly demonized for much of the twentieth century. Where are these people when alcohol and Big Pharma are on the screen?

Television shows like HBO's *Insecure* and ABC's *Black-ish* have seamlessly integrated cannabis use into their narratives, treating it as a commonplace part of their characters' lives.

In *Insecure*, the protagonist, Issa Dee, often shares scenes with her friends where cannabis use is featured. Instead of relying on stereotypes or making it the focus of the narrative, the show portrays it as a casual, social activity. This realistic and normalized portrayal is a significant departure from previous depictions of cannabis use on television, signaling the shift in societal attitudes, particularly in Black culture.

Similarly, in *Black-ish*, the topic of cannabis is dealt with in a nuanced, thoughtful way. In one notable episode, the parents, Dre and Rainbow, have a candid discussion about cannabis after they find weed in their home. This episode explores various perspectives on cannabis use, including its recreational and medicinal uses, as well as the racial disparities in cannabis-related arrests. By dealing with these issues head-on, the show contributes to the ongoing discourse centered around the plant.

These shows are using their platforms to question the stigma associated with cannabis use, to explore its potential benefits, and to address the broader societal issues surrounding its vilification. With the increased legalization and acceptance of cannabis in many parts of the world, it's likely that we'll continue to see more of these narratives in mainstream media. This evolution not only reflects the changing attitudes toward cannabis but also helps to further normalize it as a product, fostering a more open and honest conversation about its role in society.

Documentary films like *Weed the People, The Union: The Business Behind Getting High, The Culture High,* and *Grass is Greener* offer critical and informative perspectives on cannabis, delving into its history, societal implications, and the political controversy that surrounds it.

Weed the People, for instance, presents a humanistic narrative, focusing on families seeking cannabis treatments for their children's life-threatening illnesses. It underscores the potential medical benefits of cannabis and the dire need for more comprehensive research and access.

The Union: The Business Behind Getting High dives into the underworld of the lucrative cannabis industry in British Columbia. It sheds light on the complexities of the cannabis business, discussing its growth, its impact on the economy, and the contentious policies that govern its commercialization.

The Culture High, a sequel to *The Union,* takes a broader look at the global perception of cannabis. It explores the ongoing War on Drugs, the societal impacts of cannabis prohibition, and the cultural shift toward cannabis acceptance, showcasing interviews with celebrities, former undercover agents, and university professors.

Grass is Greener, a Netflix original documentary, presents an analysis of the complex relationship between cannabis and American society. It delves into the racialized history of cannabis legislation and the stark disparities in cannabis-related arrests and incarceration. The film also explores the cultural impact of cannabis, especially within the music and entertainment industries.

Murder Mountain is a Netflix documentary series that delves into the dark and often misunderstood world of Humboldt County, California, a region infamous for its rogue cannabis production. The series focuses on the disappearance of 29-year-old Garret Rodriguez and uncovers a web of crime, corruption, and cannabis in the Emerald Triangle. Through interviews with locals, law enforcement, and family members, it paints a complex picture of a community caught between the lucrative but lawless old ways and the challenges of legitimization in the era of cannabis legalization. The series blends true crime and social commentary, highlighting the deep-rooted issues surrounding the American dream gone awry.

These documentaries serve as valuable educational tools, challenging preconceived notions and misinformation about cannabis. By highlighting different aspects of cannabis—from its medical use and business potential to its cultural significance, the social injustices tied to its prohibition, and the twisted sides of the illicit market—these films contribute to a more nuanced and informed dialogue about cannabis in our society. They represent a key component of the evolving narrative, paving the way for more informed and open discussions about the plant's role in our world.

Roll Up for Equity, a documentary film I am currently directing and producing, is in the making as we speak. As a team we aim to provide a comprehensive and accurate portrayal of what it takes to be an activist and mobilize a community toward an equitable cannabis industry despite the many hurdles experienced while navigating the ever-changing landscape and government officials who are reluctant to change. There are multiple layers to this rapidly-evolving sector, and the film promises to present a holistic perspective. Roll Up for Equity exposes San Diego's struggle for social equity within its regulated cannabis industry, highlighting passionate local advocates pushing for accountability and change in America's Finest City.

My purpose as a filmmaker is to expose the heart of the cannabis industry by showcasing the opportunities and challenges that define its uniqueness. My films present firsthand accounts from a diverse range of industry players, including growers, processors, retailers, and advocates. I strive to give the viewer a front row seat at understanding our struggles, and victories while carving our own paths within this complex business environment.

Historically the cannabis plant has been widely stigmatized and demonized due to the various political, cultural, and societal factors we have discussed throughout this book. Needless to say, up until not too long ago, there were very few resources discussing cannabis unbiasedly in mainstream culture. As activists became more vocal a few reliable sources began to appear divulging information about cannabis and its use, while the mainstream media often portrayed it in a negative light. Cannabis consumption was mostly hidden and done in secret, and there was a prevailing narrative that linked it to crime, laziness, and moral decay.

High Times magazine, founded by Tom Forçade in 1974, has had an enormous influence on cannabis culture over the past several decades. Initially created as a one-off spoof of Playboy, complete with a centerfold of a cannabis plant, High Times quickly developed into a serious publication that played a significant role in shaping and promoting cannabis culture in the United States and beyond.

The magazine became an essential platform for cannabis enthusiasts and advocates, featuring articles on cultivation techniques, strain reviews, and the legal and political issues surrounding cannabis. It also showcased a countercultural perspective and was known for its celebrity interviews and coverage of music and lifestyle topics. Furthermore, High Times was one of the first national publications to provide a space for open and honest discussion about the use and benefits of cannabis, pushing against the prevailing stigmas of the time.

Over the years, High Times has played a significant role in influencing perceptions around cannabis. During an era when mainstream media often demonized cannabis and those who used it, High Times took a radically different approach, celebrating cannabis and advocating for its legalization.

High Times also launched the Cannabis Cup in 1988, an annual competition that became the most prestigious award event in the cannabis industry. The Cannabis Cup helped to raise standards in cannabis cultivation and has promoted the development of new and improved cultivars. The magazine has faced challenges as attitudes and laws around cannabis have shifted. The rise of the internet, the increasing acceptance of cannabis in mainstream culture, and the magazine's internal changes in leadership have caused major highs and lows that I am sure deserve an entire book to explore. However, the magazine has seemingly adapted as it is still around, and it is now involved in the complex world of legal cannabis retail in California. The magazine has also continued hosting its legacy events worldwide.

In the digital age, the internet and social media platforms have become instrumental in shaping perceptions of cannabis. These platforms serve as forums for sharing information, discussing policy reform, and normalizing cannabis in wellness, lifestyle, culture, and business. Websites like Leafly, for instance, provide a wealth of information about different cannabis strains, effects, brands, and local dispensaries. They also publish news and stories on various cannabis-related topics, contributing to public education and influencing the perception of cannabis.

Similarly to Leafly, Weedmaps is a popular online marketplace for cannabis products, serving as a comprehensive resource for consumers and businesses alike. Founded in 2008, the platform provides detailed information about cannabis dispensaries, delivery services, and cannabis brands. Users can browse products, read reviews, and even place orders for pickup or delivery, depending on local laws. With its extensive database, Weedmaps has become a platform that connects consumers to cannabis businesses. Both Leafly and Weedmaps are examples of ancillary cannabis businesses. They are more than media companies; they consider themselves tech companies and do not touch the plant.

One of my favorite platforms to read information about the cannabis industry is Beard Bros Media. Beard Bros Media is a renowned platform for cannabis-related news and analysis, delivering valuable insights from the vantage point of industry insiders. They provide the audience with in-depth, up-to-date information on the cannabis space.

Known for their robust reporting and nuanced analysis, Beard Bros Media is the go-to source for a wide range of individuals, from cannabis enthusiasts and patients, to entrepreneurs and investors seeking insight into the industry's trends and developments. Beard Bros Media covers a spectrum of topics that include current events, legislation changes, medical advancements, tech innovations, market trends, and cultural developments.

What sets Beard Bros Media apart is their industry insider's perspective. Their team consists of experienced professionals who have their fingers on the pulse of the industry, because they are fully immersed in the cannabis space as an organization. This allows them to provide unique and informed insights that go beyond surface-level reporting. I have been following them since 2019 and can attest to how they get into complex issues, offering analysis that helps the public to understand the broader implications of the cannabis space.

Moreover, Beard Bros Media actively champions the therapeutic potential of cannabis and the broader movement toward legalization. They use their platform not only to inform but also to advocate for a more progressive, equitable, and sustainable cannabis industry. In a landscape filled with misinformation and stigma, Beard Bros Media stands as a trusted source of reliable, insightful, and forward-thinking cannabis journalism. Their commitment to delivering high-quality information and analysis from an insider's perspective truly distinguishes them in the cannabis media space.

Another great resource is Sens Culture Magazine, a publication based in Puerto Rico. Sens Culture holds a prominent position in the realm of the Latinx cannabis culture. The magazine provides a vibrant platform to explore and promote the various facets of cannabis, offering a unique blend of inclusive educational articles, personal narratives, and in-depth analyses of cannabis-related topics. By pushing the boundaries of conventional discourse and shedding light on the dynamic, ever-evolving world of cannabis, Sens Culture Magazine has positioned itself at the cutting edge of cannabis culture in the Caribbean and in Latin America. This resource serves not just as a touchpoint for those within the community, but as an essential guide for anyone looking to understand the complexities of cannabis.

There are several media organizations dedicated to cannabis news that cater to different languages and regions in addition to *High Times*, *Beard Bros Media*, and *Sens Culture Magazine*, here are a few more examples:

- *El Planteo*: Provides Spanish-language coverage of cannabis news, political developments, culture, and lifestyle.
- *Marijuana Business Daily*: This is a leading source of financial, legal, and business news for the cannabis industry. It provides valuable insights for entrepreneurs, investors, and professionals in the cannabis business.
- *Dope Magazine*: A leading publication that explores the diverse world of cannabis culture, industry trends, and lifestyle. Recognized as a credible source, the magazine covers a wide range of topics, including strain reviews, and cultivation advice.
- *San Diego Cannabis Times*: This publication covers the flourishing scene of dispensaries and cultivators in San Diego, highlighting the vibrant cannabis community within the 619, 858, and 760 area codes in California.
- *Cannabis Now*: An online and print publication, *Cannabis Now* focuses on the latest news, political developments, and health information related to cannabis.
- *Merry Jane*: Founded by rapper Snoop Dogg, *Merry Jane* covers a wide range of cannabis-related content, from news and politics to lifestyle and food.
- *Honeysuckle Magazine*: A contemporary digital and print publication that delves into progressive culture, with a unique focus on social justice, sustainability, and the evolving conversation around cannabis.

- *Hanf Magazine*: For German-speaking audiences, *Hanf Magazine* provides news and articles related to cannabis, including its medical, social, and legal aspects.
- *Dolce Vita*: This is an Italian online magazine that provides information about cannabis in various sectors, including medicine, industry, and lifestyle.

On social media platforms like Instagram, cannabis companies and influencers share cannabis-related content, from photos of different strains and products to educational posts about cannabis consumption. Reddit hosts numerous cannabis-focused communities where users can ask questions, share experiences, and discuss cannabis-related topics.

Since we are on the topic of social media, I think it behooves us to discuss the challenges the cannabis industry faces when it comes to these platforms. The rise of the cannabis industry has been accompanied by unique challenges, especially in the realm of social media marketing. Despite the increasing legalization and acceptance of cannabis across various jurisdictions, many social media platforms still impose restrictions on promoting cannabis related content. I get it, it's due to their historically illicit nature and the ongoing federal illegality in the United States. But there are ways to find out if a business is a legal entity and when the algorithm goes haywire, cannabis businesses should have a fair review as a lot of content that gets flagged might be educational in nature. I know I briefly mentioned the topic in chapter 6, nonetheless, I would like to get a little more granular in posing the challenges cannabis stakeholders experience when it comes to social media:

Major social media platforms like Meta, Instagram, Twitter, TikTok, and Snapchat have stringent policies against advertising "controlled substances," and this includes regulated adult-use and medicinal cannabis. Even in regions where cannabis is legal, companies, influencers, educators, and advocates alike are generally barred from posting on their feed and or running paid promotional campaigns. This severely limits the reach of cannabis information and makes it harder for them to attract new audiences.

In line with their advertising policies, social media platforms regularly monitor for and penalize the promotion of cannabis. Even a simple post featuring cannabis products or paraphernalia can lead to a warning, temporary account suspension, or even permanent deletion. This creates a precarious situation for cannabis companies, influencers, educators, and advocates who risk losing their entire social media presence and follower base without warning. This happens daily.

With cannabis laws varying greatly around the world and even within the same country, cannabis businesses face the challenge of tailoring their social media content to different regions. A post that is perfectly legal and acceptable in one place might violate laws or platform policies in another. This requires companies, influencers, educators, and advocates to be continually aware and considerate of the diverse legal landscapes in which their followers reside.

Due to the inability to run traditional ad campaigns, cannabis companies, influencers, educators, and advocates often struggle to measure the return on investment (ROI) for their social media efforts. Without the use of paid advertising and its accompanying analytics, it can be challenging to accurately track metrics like customer/audience acquisition costs and conversion rates.

While attitudes toward cannabis are changing, stigma and misinformation persist. This can lead to negative comments or backlash on social media, which can harm a stakeholder's reputation. Therefore, cannabis companies, influencers, educators, and advocates must not only promote but also educate their audience and combat harmful stereotypes.

If you read my first published book, The Successful Cannapreneur, you should know that I am a solutions-based mindset individual. For that reason, I have to add that despite these challenges, many cannabis stakeholders have found ways to leverage social media effectively. Content marketing, influencer partnerships, and community building are all strategies that may bypass traditional advertising restrictions (...emphasis on _may_).

Instead of directly promoting products or information, many cannabis stakeholders focus on creating valuable, engaging content for their audience. This can range from educational content about the benefits and proper usage of cannabis to behind-the-scenes showcase of the cultivation and production processes. High-quality, informative content can attract and retain followers, build brand authority, and drive sales.

Partnering with influencers is another effective way to reach a larger audience on social media. By choosing influencers who align with their brand values, cannabis companies can tap into an established audience and gain credibility through the influencer's endorsement. However, it's crucial to ensure that the influencer is aware of and adheres to all platform policies and legal regulations regarding the promotion of products.

One of the most powerful aspects of social media is its ability to foster communities. Cannabis companies can use their platforms to engage with their followers, answer questions, solicit feedback, and create a sense of belonging. This not only helps build a loyal customer base but also allows companies to position themselves as more than just a seller of products, but as a contributing member of the broader cannabis culture and community.

While social media marketing poses unique challenges for cannabis, with creativity and strategic thinking, it's possible to build a strong, engaging social media presence that respects platform policies and regulations. As societal attitudes and laws continue to evolve, we can likely expect the social media landscape for cannabis marketing to change in tandem.

Memes have played a significant role in shaping the public perception and culture of cannabis. They've served as a form of grassroots marketing, helping to normalize and destigmatize cannabis use to some extent. Through humor and relatability, memes often touch on the various aspects of cannabis culture, from the ritual of smoking and the experience of being "high," to the politics of legalization and the stereotypes often associated with users. By making these topics approachable and shareable, memes contribute to a wider public discourse, opening up conversations that might otherwise be taboo or stigmatized.

Moreover, memes have also become a way for the cannabis community to share knowledge, experiences, and even critiques of current laws and regulations. This fosters a sense of community and shared understanding among cannabis users and advocates. However, while memes can help to normalize cannabis use, they can also perpetuate stereotypes and misinformation, so their impact is complex and multifaceted.

One of my all-time favorite memes is the "Hits Blunt" meme. These memes are popular on the internet and social media. They have a format that typically features a photograph or drawing of a person who appears to be under the influence of cannabis, accompanied by a thought-provoking or paradoxical question or statement. The idea is to humorously capture the kind of "deep" or silly thoughts people claim to have after smoking cannabis. These memes often touch on philosophy, language quirks, or random observations about everyday life. The format has been widely circulated and has spawned many variations. the Hits Blunt meme is often used for comedic purposes, it also plays into stereotypes about cannabis use.

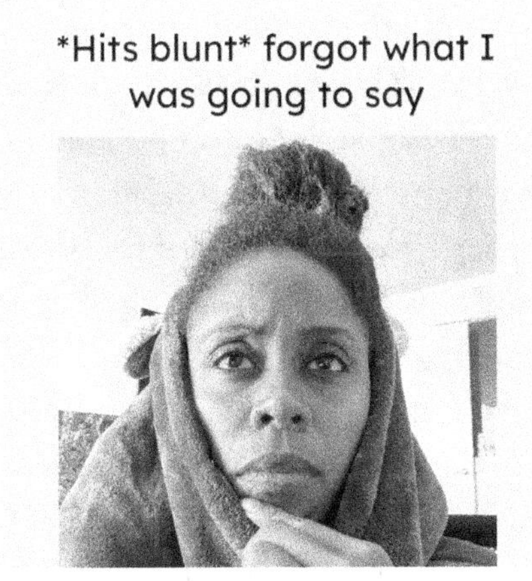

Radio and podcasts have provided another avenue for cannabis discussion and education. Traditional radio shows have been joined by a plethora of podcasts focusing on various aspects of cannabis. *Marijuana Today*, for example, brings experts together to discuss the latest developments in marijuana business and politics. "The Hash" dives into cannabis-related stories concerning science, culture, and social justice. Such platforms not only help spread reliable information about cannabis but also engage audiences in ongoing debates about its legal, economic, and health-related implications.

Mainstream podcasts like Mike Tyson's *Hotboxin'* and The *Joe Rogan Experience* have significantly contributed to the conversation around cannabis and psychedelics, shedding light on these topics for a broad audience.

Hotboxin' is co-hosted by boxing legend Mike Tyson and his co-host, Eben Britton. In the show, they engage in candid conversations with a range of guests — from celebrities to athletes, and from musicians to inspiring individuals, in Tyson's personal cannabis ranch. The discussions often venture into Tyson's personal experiences with cannabis and psychedelics, bringing a unique perspective to the table.

Similarly, *The Joe Rogan Experience*, hosted by comedian, actor, and martial artist Joe Rogan, is known for its free-form, long-form conversations that cover a wide array of topics, including cannabis and psychedelics. Rogan's candidness about his own experiences and the intellectual curiosity he brings to these discussions have helped to destigmatize and normalize the conversation around these substances. He often brings in experts from diverse fields — scientists, authors, activists, and researchers to dive deeper into these topics, fostering a dialogue based on curiosity. Rogan has had prominent figures like Elon Musk, as guests consuming cannabis on camera.

These podcasts have used their mainstream appeal to create a platform for discussing topics that have historically been considered taboo or fringe. By bringing in experts, sharing personal experiences, and engaging in open-minded discussions, they've managed to broaden public understanding and challenge preconceived notions about cannabis and psychedelics. They've played a significant role in fostering an ongoing dialogue and in slowly shifting societal attitudes toward these substances.

The growing acceptance of cannabis has made its way into academia, with numerous institutions offering courses on topics such as cannabis science, policy, business, and law. For instance, the University of Vermont offers a professional certificate in cannabis science and medicine, while the University of Maryland offers a master's in medical cannabis science and therapeutics. It's fascinating to see how even Ivy League institutions like the Yale School of Medicine are embracing cannabis research. Their newly established Center for the Science of Cannabis and Cannabinoids underscores the growing interest in understanding the full spectrum of cannabis's effects.

Researchers at Yale claim to be searching for evidence of the therapeutic applications of cannabis through rigorous scientific methods, such as double-blind, randomized, placebo-controlled studies. I believe this approach ensures a high level of accuracy in the findings, allowing for a comprehensive assessment of the plant's potential benefits.

The center isn't solely focused on the positive aspects. It is also investigating the potential harmful consequences of cannabis use. If balanced, this approach is essential for providing a nuanced and evidence-based understanding of cannabis, which is particularly important in a time when cannabis is gaining both medical and recreational acceptance.

In addition to traditional academia, a growing number of online and in-real-life education platforms now offer comprehensive training on cannabis, catering to those interested in gaining a deeper understanding of the plant and the industry. Here are a few notable examples:

- *Oaksterdam University*: Known as America's first cannabis college, Oaksterdam University provides quality training for the cannabis industry. Their courses cover a broad range of topics such as horticulture, business, law, and patient relations. They offer both in-person classes at their Oakland campus and online courses.

- *Green Flower Media:* This online platform offers a series of video-based classes led by cannabis experts. The topics range from the basics of cannabis to business operations, medical applications, growing, and cooking with cannabis. They also provide certification courses for those seeking more formal recognition of their cannabis education.
- *Cannabis Training University:* This online cannabis education platform offers a range of courses designed for beginners to advanced learners. They cover topics like cannabis laws and regulations, cultivation, cooking, extraction, and the medical uses of cannabis.
- *Clover Leaf University:* Accredited by the Colorado Department of Higher Education, Clover Leaf offers a variety of cannabis-specific courses. They provide training in areas like cultivation, cannabis law, dispensary operations, and infused product manufacturing.
- *THC University:* This platform offers online certification programs for a variety of cannabis disciplines. Their programs include growing, cannabis business, budtending, and more.

These educational platforms provide training for those interested in joining the cannabis industry or those just looking to enhance their understanding of the emerging space. As the industry continues to grow and evolve, the importance of this kind of education will simultaneously increase.

Books have played a crucial role in spreading information and shaping public opinion about cannabis. From grow guides and cookbooks to scientific research and personal memoirs, there is a wealth of literature available that caters to every aspect of cannabis interest.

For those interested in the history and politics of cannabis, books like *The Emperor Wears No Clothes*, by Jack Herer or *Smoke Signals*, by Martin A. Lee are essential reads. Those looking to grow their own cannabis might turn to *Marijuana Horticulture: The Indoor/Outdoor Medical Grower's Bible*, by Jorge Cervantes. Cookbooks like *Bong Appétit*, by the editors of MUNCHIES offer recipes for cannabis-infused dishes, reflecting the growing interest in edibles and non-smokable cannabis.

These books, along with countless others, contribute to a comprehensive body of knowledge and available information on cannabis. Furthermore, women authors in cannabis have made significant contributions to the broad and multifaceted dialogue surrounding cannabis. With their work, women's perspectives and voices continue to contribute to the evolution in the perception of cannabis from a stigmatized substance to an acknowledged aspect of our culture and economy. Below are a few books written by women authors I admire:

- *The Successful Canna-preneur*, by me, JM Balbuena: This book provides a realistic perspective on what it takes to achieve success in the legal cannabis industry. It offers a comprehensive exploration of the cannabis industry's opportunities and challenges and provides the reader with a formula to keep a solution-based mindset while navigating a new and restricted industry.
- *How to Succeed in the Cannabis Industry*, by Dasheeda Dawson: Dawson provides readers with a roadmap for success in the booming cannabis industry. Drawing from her own experiences, she offers insights into the industry's landscape and shares valuable advice for those looking to enter or already navigating the cannabis sector.
- *Women & Weed*, by Elena Frankel: Frankel's book focuses on the intersection of women and cannabis culture, exploring the role and impact of women in the industry. It addresses the therapeutic benefits of cannabis for women and provides a platform for the voices and experiences of women within the cannabis community.

- *Weed Mom*, by Danielle Simone Brand: In this book, Brand uncovers the world of mothers who consume cannabis. She breaks down the stigma and stereotypes associated with cannabis use and parenting, providing a candid exploration of what it means to be a "weed mom."
- *A Woman's Guide to Cannabis*, by Nikki Furrer: Furrer's guidebook demystifies cannabis for women. It provides helpful information on using cannabis for health, wellness, and relaxation, covering topics like dosage, delivery methods, and strains.

Each of these books brings a unique perspective to the conversation around cannabis, be it from an entrepreneurial, gendered, parental, or medicinal viewpoint. They collectively form a rich, diverse body of knowledge that informs, educates, and inspires readers, further advancing the understanding and acceptance of cannabis in our society.

In the world of cannabis, events aren't just gatherings; they're an essential part of the culture that engages all senses. These occasions give the cannabis community the unique opportunity to "test" products in real-time, creating a level of trust between consumers and brands that online interactions can seldom achieve. Moreover, they attract the true connoisseurs, those who deeply appreciate the plant in all its forms and uses. Such events serve as fertile ground for building personal connections, and for many, cannabis is a deeply intimate experience that resonates at a unique frequency in each user. This bond fosters innovation and advocacy within the cannabis industry, offering a chance for all stakeholders, from growers to retailers, and from newcomers to seasoned consumers, to strengthen their ties within the growing community.

In an era where the legalization of cannabis is gaining widespread regulatory support and its adoption into the mainstream consumer market is growing, events that capture these multi-sensory, personal experiences are more important than ever. For small businesses seeking longevity and impact, these authentic relationships built in communal spaces are invaluable. As we look toward the future, events that truly encapsulate these elements could very well set the standard for how the cannabis industry engages with its community.

Events like Spannabis, Hall of Flowers, MJBiz Con, Cannabisalud, San Diego's Farmers Cup, and the Emerald Cup serve as examples of what cannabis culture can offer in a communal space. Each event has its own unique flavor, yet they all share a common purpose: to bring together diverse members of the cannabis community for collaboration, education, and celebration of the plant they love.

Spannabis, based in Spain, is one of Europe's largest cannabis events, encompassing not only a trade show but also seminars and even a cannabis film festival. Hall of Flowers, on the other hand, focuses on the B2B aspect of cannabis, providing a stage for emerging brands to showcase their products to retailers, investors, and media. MJBiz Con and Cannabisalud put together gatherings that lean more toward the corporate, commerce, and ancillary aspects of the industry, with work-shops, lectures, and exhibits by industry experts appealing to the busi-ness-side of cannabis.

San Diego's Farmers Cup and the Emerald Cup, for instance, both veer more into the connoisseur side of things. These events feature competitions that crown the best quality cannabis, judged on various criteria such as potency, flavor, and overall experience. They also offer live entertainment and a platform for artisanal growers to showcase their craft to the community.

The diversity of events in cannabis is a vivid reflection of its multifaceted community members. Among these gatherings, women-centric events stand out as empowering platforms for women entrepre-neurs, consumers, and advocates in the cannabis industry. Networking opportunities, workshops, and discussions led by influential women are common features at events like the yearly Higher Conference in Phil-adelphia, PA, a conference for Women of Color and supporters.

Then there are culinary experiences, an oasis for foodies and culi-nary artists. Chefs specializing in cannabis-infused cuisine often take the stage to offer cooking classes, tasting events, and gastronomic fairs, offering an exciting fusion of culinary arts and cannabis science.

Holistic experiences go a step further by integrating cannabis into yoga and meditation sessions. These events offer attendees the unique opportunity to deepen their mindfulness and relaxation techniques by pairing them with the benefits of cannabis. In a similar manner, wellness events concentrate on the medicinal aspects of cannabis. Here, you can find wellness professionals, therapists, and researchers discussing the therapeutic uses of cannabinoids for sleep, mental health, pain management, and more.

Educational events serve as informative platforms designed to enlighten the public or specific groups on the many aspects of cannabis. These events often feature lecture series, 101 classes, and scientific symposia to provide accurate and updated information, dispelling myths, and misconceptions about the plant.

Career fairs in the cannabis sector are becoming more commonplace as well. As the industry expands, these events offer a valuable space for job seekers to connect with companies seeking new talent, offering a vital avenue for those aiming to start a career in this burgeoning field.

Rounding off the spectrum of cannabis-related events are those that focus on lifestyle and culture. These gatherings celebrate the broader societal aspects of cannabis, including art exhibitions, music festivals, and even fashion shows.

These events illustrate the vast spectrum of interests within the cannabis community, from the business-oriented to the activist, the casual consumer, and the dedicated grower. Yet, despite these differences, they share the power to bring people together through their shared passion for the plant. Such events contribute to the strengthening of the community bonds that are so vital for the continued evolution of cannabis in broader society.

As the global perspective on cannabis undergoes a massive overhaul, the sports world is not far behind in reevaluating its stance on the plant. From the iconic Olympic swimmer Michael Phelps to emerging stars like Sha'Carri Richardson, the intersection of cannabis and sports has sparked both controversy and change. Major leagues such as the Major League Baseball (MLB) and the National Basketball Association (NBA) have modified their cannabis policies, either by decriminalizing its use or by adjusting testing protocols, signaling a more forthcoming approach to the substance. The evolving relationship between athletes and cannabis, involves more than just high-profile cases and headlines. It also about how major sports leagues are rethinking their policies. Whether it's for medicinal purposes or recreational use, the leafy green plant is undeniably a player in the arena of sports, spawning conversations with the potential to redefine athlete wellness.

High-profile athletes like Michael Phelps, Sha'Carri Richardson, and Chris Webber have been embroiled in controversies or business ventures surrounding cannabis, further intensifying the debate:

Michael Phelps, the most decorated Olympian of all time, faced backlash after a photograph of him smoking a bong emerged in 2009. Although he didn't face suspension from international competition, the incident sparked a debate on whether cannabis actually has a place in sports, given that it's not a performance-enhancing drug in the traditional sense.

Sha'Carri Richardson, an American sprinter, became the center of a similar debate when she was suspended for one month after testing positive for THC in 2021. Her suspension led to her missing the Tokyo Olympics and initiated a wider conversation about the stringent anticannabis policies within the sports world, particularly since she had used cannabis in a legal state and for reported emotional distress.

Brittney Griner, a center for the Phoenix Mercury in the WNBA, also played for overseas leagues during the American league's off-season to supplement her income. In recent years, she was a part of UMMC Ekaterinburg, a Russian basketball club owned by oligarch Iskander Makhmudov, which has a long-standing relationship with her US-based team. Griner was apprehended at a Russian airport for carrying cannabis upon her return to rejoin the Russian team. She claimed the cannabis was mistakenly packed in her bag and her defense pointed out that she had a medical cannabis card recommended by a doctor in Arizona for managing injuries acquired through years of athletic competition. However, Russian law bans cannabis possession under any conditions, similarly to US federal regulations. Recently, Griner was convicted in Russia on charges of drug possession and smuggling, receiving a nine-year prison sentence. The case became politically charged, culminating in a significant prisoner exchange between the US and Russia.

Ricky Williams, a talented National Football League (NFL) running back, had a career fraught with controversies largely due to his use of cannabis, which led to several suspensions and financial penalties under the league's stringent substance abuse policy at the time. Williams took the bold step of retiring prematurely to escape the constant scrutiny, only to stage a remarkable comeback later. Beyond his on-field exploits, Williams has become a vocal advocate for the responsible use of cannabis, particularly emphasizing its potential benefits for mental well-being and pain management. Despite the challenges and setbacks he faced, including jeopardizing a promising athletic career, Williams has turned his experience into a platform to educate others about the medicinal and therapeutic potential of cannabis. He argues that the plant can offer a safer, more natural alternative to conventional treatments for mental health issues and chronic pain, a message he continues to spread in various advocacy roles today.

Nick Diaz is an American professional boxer and mixed martial artist who has been suspended multiple times by the Nevada State Athletic Commission for testing positive for cannabis metabolites. Diaz has been vocal about his cannabis use, questioning the substance's banned status in the sport.

In the MLB, Tim Lincecum, a pitcher, was cited for cannabis possession in 2009. While this incident didn't result in a suspension, it did make headlines and added to the ongoing discussion about cannabis in professional sports. While Tyrann Mathieu, also known as the "Honey Badger," faced disciplinary action while playing college football for LSU due to cannabis use. Fortunately for him, this did not prevent him from becoming a professional player in the NFL.

Kyle Turley, a former NFL offensive lineman, has become an outspoken advocate for the use of cannabis in the sports world, particularly as an alternative to opioids for managing pain and other health issues. His journey to advocacy was fueled by personal experience, as he struggled with chronic pain, mental health issues, and the side effects of pharmaceutical drugs during and after his football career. Turley has often spoken about how cannabis not only helped him manage his symptoms but also significantly improved his quality of life.

After retiring from the NFL, Turley founded a cannabis company focused on providing CBD products, championing them as a safer, more natural option for pain management and mental wellness. He's been quite vocal about his belief that cannabis can save lives by reducing the dependence on addictive and potentially harmful pharmaceuticals, a claim that resonates with many athletes who face similar challenges. Turley also engages in public speaking and participates in advocacy efforts aimed at changing the policies surrounding cannabis use in professional sports and beyond.

I had the pleasure to collaborate with Kyle Turley at a cannabis event we put together in 2018 at his alma mater, San Diego State University (SDSU). Cannabis 4 The Cause was SDSU's first-ever educational cannabis event. We had a great line-up of speakers discussing cannabis in sports injuries and veterans' health and wellness. Turley, who played offensive tackle, was named an All-American in his senior year, was a first-round draft pick and two-time All-Pro in the NFL.

During the Cannabis 4 The Cause event, he shared his story and advised that the number one issue facing NFL football players is Chronic Traumatic Encephalopathy (CTE). CTE is a progressive degenerative brain disorder that can happen in people with a history of repeated blows to the head, often sustained while playing contact sports such as football or boxing. During his presentation, Turley informed us that he believes cannabis to be the only remedy currently available that helps to heal the physical tissue in the brain naturally, as cannabinoids have neuroprotectants and antioxidants.

Chris Webber, a retired NBA player, has taken a different route. Instead of becoming a cautionary tale on the field, he's walking the grueling path of entrepreneurship in the regulated cannabis industry. In 2021, at the peak of the pandemic, Webber co-founded a $100 million private equity cannabis fund to invest in cannabis companies from underserved communities. As of today, the Social Equity Impact Ventures, which includes Chris Webber and businesswoman Lavetta Willis, has been named by the Dormitory Authority of the State of New York (DASNY) as the entity that will manage the massive public-private fund meant to bring equity to the state's cannabis industry.

Many eyebrows have been raised given that, as of today (September 2023), there is no evidence of the capital being raised or any social equity candidates receiving financial assistance from this venture. However, let's not forget this is cannabis; people may come in with good intentions, but things usually take much longer to unfold. This industry is not for the faint of heart and does not discriminate, even if you're a "Hall of Famer."

The intersection of cannabis culture with sports and entertainment continues to evolve, as evidenced by NBA Hall-of-Famer Dwyane Wade's recent collaboration with Jeeter, a popular preroll cannabis brand. This partnership not only commemorates Wade's illustrious basketball career but also signals a broader cultural acceptance of cannabis within professional sports communities.

In August 2023, Wade released an exclusive product called "Hall of Flame," a limited-edition Jeeter box that features three infused joints, also known as Jeeter Baby Cannons. According to the press, the branding and collaboration concept is a nod to Wade's basketball legacy, capturing the essence of who he was as a player and celebrating his journey into the next phase of his life. Available in three fully legal states, this venture represents a significant moment not just for Wade and Jeeter but for the cannabis industry as a whole. It emphasizes the changing perceptions surrounding cannabis use, highlighting its transition from a stigmatized plant to a product embraced by high-profile public figures, including athletes.

Various sports organizations have been reassessing their stance on cannabis, especially considering the changing legal status, and increased societal acceptance. Currently, their rules vary widely from one organization to another, and we can bet on the fact that these rules are to adjust in tandem with the evolution of legal status of cannabis.

Take the MLB for example. The organization took a definitive step by removing cannabis from its list of "drugs of abuse" in December 2019. The league now treats cannabis similarly to alcohol, meaning players can still be fined for activities involving its possession or distribution but won't face suspension merely for testing positive. Meanwhile, the NBA, amid the extraordinary circumstances of the COVID-19 pandemic, suspended its random cannabis testing for the 2020–2021 season. This change became permanent, signaling professional sports' openness to reevaluating its stance on cannabis in the US.

The National Football League (NFL) has also softened its policies. With the 2020 collective bargaining agreement, the NFL specified that players would no longer face suspension for testing positive for cannabis. Moreover, the testing period was restricted to just the first two weeks of training camp, and the threshold for a positive result was raised, making it less likely for players to be penalized. The National Hockey League (NHL) has its own specific approach. While it doesn't list cannabis as a banned substance, it does test for it. Should a player be found with a "dangerously high level" of THC, they could be referred to the league's Substance Abuse and Behavioral Health Program for further evaluation.

In a similar manner, the Ultimate Fighting Championship (UFC) announced in January 2021 that testing positive for THC would no longer be considered a violation unless it could be proven that the substance was used for performance enhancement. Even the World Anti-Doping Agency (WADA) has made adjustments. Cannabis remains on WADA's list of prohibited substances, but the threshold for a positive test was raised in 2013 to minimize out-of-competition positive results that have no direct correlation to an athlete's performance.

The worldwide sports arena is increasingly embracing cannabis. In 2023, cbdMD, a prominent CBD company, secured an exclusive sponsorship deal with Club Sport Herediano, a FIFA-affiliated professional soccer team in Costa Rica. This groundbreaking partnership stands as the sole collaboration between a CBD brand and a FIFA-recognized premier division professional soccer team.

Collectively, these changes reflect an evolving perspective on cannabis in the world of professional sports, with leagues and governing bodies increasingly acknowledging the complexities surrounding its use.

"It's the NBA, man. Everybody does it, to be honest. It's like wine at this point." (Kevin Durant, bbc.com)

The influence of cannabis on the culinary arts is as vibrant as the flavors chefs are crafting with this versatile herb. In a landscape where cannabis is transitioning from taboo to table fare, the culinary world is getting a taste of something groundbreaking. This ascension didn't happen overnight. The origins of cannabis-infused edibles trace back to pioneers like Brownie Mary, a.k.a. Mary Jane Rathbun, who used her cannabis-infused brownies as a form of medical relief for AIDS and cancer patients in the 1980s. Her work not only offered a compassionate solution to those in need but also opened the door for cannabis to be considered a viable ingredient in the kitchen.

Over time, cannabis has moved from brownies on a bake sale table to gourmet kitchens. Specialized chefs like Amanda Jackson are bringing legitimacy and flair to cannabis-infused dining. Trained at Johnson & Wales University and boasting over two decades of professional experience, Chef Jackson doesn't merely aim to serve edibles that get you high; she aims to enhance the culinary experience itself with cannabis as a foundational ingredient. Since embarking on her own business venture in 2017, she has been revolutionizing how we understand and enjoy cannabis as an ingredient, incorporating it thoughtfully into dishes that stand alone for their flavor profiles, textures, and overall dining experience.

Cannabis cuisine has also made its way into mainstream media, taking the food world by storm. Programs like "Bong Appetite," "Chopped 420," and "Cooked with Cannabis" are elevating cannabis-infused cooking to an art form, showcasing on platforms like the Food Network and various streaming services. These shows are demystifying cannabis cuisine, guiding the public through the intricacies of cooking with cannabis and making it accessible for foodies, home cooks, and professional chefs alike.

Even fast-food chains are getting in on the action. The collaboration between Jack in the Box and Weedmaps signaled a new era where cannabis is not only accepted but celebrated in mainstream culinary circles. This crossover collaboration made headlines, pointing to a future where cannabis could have a common place in personal and commercial kitchens as any other herb or spice, and I'm here for it!

In this culinary revolution, cannabis is more than a psychoactive substance; it is a versatile ingredient contributing to gastronomic creativity and innovation. By blending the traditional with the groundbreaking, the culinary world is setting the stage for a cannabis-infused future that promises to delight the senses in new and exciting ways.

On the other side of entertainment, the relationship between cannabis and music is deeply intertwined, a long-standing liaison that dates back to at least the Jazz Age of the 1920s as we explored a couple of chapters ago. Both culturally and lyrically, this plant has found its way into the heart of various musical movements, from jazz to hip-hop to rock and beyond. Artists often use their platforms to sing praises of the euphoria, relaxation, or inspiration they find in cannabis, weaving this once-taboo subject into the fabric of the world's music history.

Take, for instance, the 1934 song "Sweet Marihuana" sung by Gertrude Michael in the movie *Murder at the Vanities*. In a bold move for its time, the song unabashedly glorified the plant. The jazz era, particularly in Black communities in the US, saw widespread cannabis consumption, often referred to in slang like "grass" or "reefer." As discussed in an earlier chapter, jazz legends like Louis Armstrong even had their own terms for it; Armstrong called it "the gage" and considered it a form of medicine that fueled his artistry. Songs like Cab Calloway's "Reefer Man" became anthems of the era, encapsulating the relationship between cannabis and the flourishing jazz scene.

The influence of cannabis in music didn't stop with jazz; it found a new home with the Beat Poets and spoken word artists of the 1950s and '60s, whose writings and performances were deeply entwined with their experiences with the plant. When the cultural tides turned toward rock and roll, cannabis followed. The Beatles, who were introduced to cannabis by Bob Dylan in 1964, subtly incorporated its influences into songs like "Got to Get You into My Life."

When discussing the interplay between cannabis and music, it's impossible to ignore the significant contributions of figures like Bob Marley and Peter Tosh. Their activism and advocacy were ahead of their time, yet their message has proven to be timeless, resonating with a new generation of artists, entrepreneurs, and consumers in the cannabis community. Bob Marley and Peter Tosh, two iconic figures in reggae music, were outspoken advocates for cannabis, or "ganja" as it is commonly referred to in Rastafarian culture, which they were a part of.

In a time when the plant was largely demonized and criminalized, Marley and Tosh used their platforms to not just celebrate its use but also to advocate for its spiritual and medicinal benefits. Their influence is felt not only in the music that pays homage to cannabis but also in the growing acceptance and decriminalization of the plant worldwide. Both Marley and Tosh have left legacies that go beyond their music; their contributions to the green renaissance have significant implications on how cannabis is perceived today.

As we moved into the era of hip-hop and rap, cannabis remained a robust influence. Dr. Dre and Snoop Dogg's iconic 1992 album *The Chronic* didn't just nod to cannabis; it embraced it as both a muse and a lifestyle. This tradition has continued into the modern era with artists like Cypress Hill, Jay-Z, Wiz Khalifa, and Kid Cudi, who not only incorporate cannabis into their lyrics but also invest in cannabis-related ventures and collaborations.

This rich history of cannabis in music serves as a mirror reflecting broader social and cultural transitions. From the jazz musicians of New Orleans to the hip-hop artists from coast to coast, cannabis has been a backdrop, a muse, and often, a focal point. Whether subtly integrated or overtly celebrated, the plant has remained a constant thread in the ever-evolving creative world, a testament to its enduring cultural relevance. Whether we're talking about Rick James's love ballad to Mary Jane, Styles P. getting high in his lyrics, D'Angelo's sultry "Brown Sugar," or Willy Nelson's subtlety in "In a Memory," the plant's essence is captured and perpetuated in the songs we sing and the music we love. It is more than a recurring theme; the plant is a character in the story of world music. A story that continues to be written today.

The symbiotic relationship between the worlds of cannabis and music through the years is most recently exemplified in the success stories of entrepreneurs who operate in both realms. Berner, the co-founder and CEO of Cookies, one of the most prominent cannabis brands and retailers, is a prime example. A hip-hop artist himself, Berner has leveraged his music career to gain unparalleled access to influential circles and audiences, subsequently benefiting his cannabis ventures.

One collaboration that came out of this intersection is Cookies's recent partnership with Grammy Award-winning artist Erykah Badu. Earlier this year, Badu released her own line of cannabis flower named "That Badu," exclusively available at Cookies. This premium line of cannabis products is specifically designed with the wellness of women in mind, showcasing how personalized and specific the industry's target marketing has become.

The collaboration serves as a testament to the influence of music artists in the burgeoning cannabis market. During her "Unfollow Me" tour, Badu promoted the brand, did meet-and-greets with fans at Cookies Stores, and even implemented engaging marketing strategies to connect with her fans through their love for her music and the herb.

These types of collaborations are an affirmation of the cultural revolution happening around cannabis, particularly as it becomes more mainstream and tailored to specific communities and needs. Both Cookies and Badu bring their distinct audiences, broadening the reach of the products and contributing to the de-stigmatization of cannabis consumption in mainstream culture.

If you have a taste for both fashion and purpose-driven merchandise, you're likely aware of the close connection between the cannabis lifestyle and making bold statements. Throughout history, the cannabis culture has made countercultural statements through clothing and accessories, creating a timeless bond. This affinity for fashion has only grown within the cannabis industry, with proud pot enthusiasts expressing their love for the plant through branded merchandise. From wearable advocacy to art, sustainability, and everything in between, cannabis companies have turned to fashion as a means to connect emotionally with their consumers.

Cannabis consumers are emerging from the shadows and openly discussing the wellness benefits of the plant in their lives. This shift can be attributed to several factors. First, worldwide legalization is on the horizon, with many parts of the world now permitting medicinal or recreational cannabis use. This surge in legality has naturally increased the demand for cannabis-inspired clothing and accessories. Second, the internet and the rise of e-commerce have made it easier than ever to access cannabis-themed fashion. In the past, acquiring such clothing often meant making it yourself or visiting a local hippie store. Now, all you need is internet connection to explore and purchase cannabis-inspired merchandise.

As the cannabis fashion industry continues to expand, expect to see a surge in new brands entering the scene. This trend is particularly evident as cannabis legalization becomes more widespread and regulations surrounding the industry become less stringent. These emerging brands will offer fresh perspectives on cannabis fashion, leading to increased competition, which is likely to keep prices reasonable and drive the popularity of this growing fashion genre. Moreover, new entrants will diversify the types of products available in the cannabis fashion market, moving beyond standard items like t-shirts and hoodies to explore innovative and unique designs.

While cannabis has always had a place in fashion, hemp has recently gained prominence as a key material in the cannabis fashion industry. Hemp fabrics are versatile and sustainable, making them ideal for creating various clothing items, including baseball caps and bags. With a wide range of textures and designs possible with hemp, this material has the potential to become even more popular in the years ahead. It's a sustainable, cost-effective, and eco-friendly option that aligns with the growing demand for environmentally conscious fashion choices.

Brands like Levi Strauss & Co. are at the forefront of incorporating hemp into their fashion lines. Levi's introduced jeans made with recycled Circulose fiber and increased the use of cottonized hemp in their products. This pioneering spirit aims to create more sustainable, eco-friendly clothing options. Hemp's advantages, such as water and chemical efficiency, make it an attractive choice for forward-thinking fashion brands. Expect more brands to follow suit and incorporate hemp into their designs.

Jungmaven, a sustainable lifestyle brand, focuses on crafting timeless, quality apparel and accessories. Known for its hemp and organic cotton pieces, this brand emphasizes durability. Jungmaven's mission is to encourage everyone to embrace hemp-based clothing. With a blend of organic cotton, the brand brings luxury and style to hemp fashion. Their efforts have contributed to the revitalization of hemp as a fashionable and eco-conscious material.

The cannabis fashion industry is on a steady rise, driven by the increasing global acceptance of the plant and the convenience of e-commerce. As the industry continues to grow, expect fresh brands, diverse products, and innovative materials like hemp to shape the future of cannabis fashion. This exciting fusion of style and culture is here to stay, celebrating a lifestyle deeply intertwined with the cannabis plant.

Cannabis has held a profound place in human history, often recognized as an entheogen, a plant capable of expanding consciousness and facilitating spiritual growth. This connection between cannabis and spirituality spans various cultures. Hindu sadhus, Zoroastrians, and Rastafarians revere cannabis as a sacred tool, and in Ayurveda, one of the world's oldest holistic healing systems, cannabis is revered as a divine healing plant closely associated with Lord Shiva. However, ancient texts like the Vedas also caution against its inappropriate or recreational use, likening it to a toxin when used without reverence.

The distinction between spiritual development and mere pleasure in the realm of cannabis can sometimes be subtle. Nevertheless, recent years have witnessed a resurgence of a more elevated approach to cannabis consumption, one that places a renewed emphasis on its spiritual significance. Across the world, people are integrating cannabis into practices such as yoga, meditation, and mindfulness. Alongside these informal affiliations, we see the emergence of semi-organized cannabis-based religions and churches, including names like the Coachella Valley Church of California and the Hawai'i Cannabis Ministry. These spiritual communities often adopt creeds that champion values like love, unity, tolerance, equality, and kindness. These spiritual practices and communities centered around cannabis revere the plant as a gateway to the divine: a means of connecting with oneself, others, and the Earth.

Recreational consumers occasionally claim spiritual insights as a byproduct of cannabis consumption. Primarily, the new wave of spiritual cannabis consumers treats the plant as a sacrament or a teacher, believing it imparts profound wisdom and messages. Before consumption, setting a clear intention becomes a vital ritual. The act of ingesting cannabis is often accompanied by a carefully designed ceremony, steeping the plant with spiritual significance.

This philosophy represents a conscious effort to counter the recent commercialization of cannabis and reconnect with its deep historical and spiritual roots. In the wake of the Green Renaissance, the mainstream world associates cannabis primarily with market shares and industry. Cannabis spirituality strives for a holistic understanding of the plant, embracing not only its therapeutic qualities but also its spiritual and transcendental aspects. Spirituality is also a part of this movement, with advocates supporting a more spiritual relationship with the plant.

In essence, there is the medical world and the adult-use world. But the evolving spiritual approach to cannabis is also significant and serves as a reclamation of its ancient, sacred qualities amid the modern-day surge in commercialization and mass consumption. It encourages all stakeholders to look beyond the plant's economic value and explore the profound spiritual wisdom it may hold.

Growing Cannabiz

The burgeoning cannabis industry has grown beyond the cultivation and sale of the plant. It now spans numerous sectors, including medicine, food and beverage, cosmetics, apparel, tourism, and more. The industry's growth has spurred innovation, with companies developing new cannabis and hemp-based products, improving cultivation techniques, and pioneering advancements in extraction and processing technologies.

Cannabis legalization has also prompted the growth of ancillary businesses. Law firms, consulting agencies, marketing companies, software developers, and more have stepped in to support cannabis businesses navigate the complex landscape of regulations, compliance, and industry trends.

According to Grand View Research, the US cannabis industry has been experiencing explosive growth, with its market value hitting $13.2 billion in 2022. The sector is expected to continue this upward trajectory, expanding at a compound annual growth rate of 14.2% between 2023 and 2030. This boom isn't just fueled by recreational or medical cannabis use; the plant's derivatives are increasingly finding their way into various other industries as well. Cannabis is becoming a versatile ingredient that crosses traditional market boundaries, signaling a sea change in how this once-stigmatized plant is perceived and utilized in the American marketplace.

Despite the size of the industry, cannabis businesses are still stigmatized. Hence, it remains a mostly cash business. The Secure and Fair Enforcement Regulation Banking Act (SAFER) stands as a significant piece of legislation designed to offer protection and stability to financial institutions engaging with state-approved cannabis businesses and their service providers. While this bill holds immense promise for the cannabis industry, it currently lingers in the Senate Committee on Banking, Housing, and Urban Affairs, where it underwent a hearing on May 11, 2023. The committee has not yet made a decision regarding the bill's progression to the full Senate, leaving the timeline and potential approval uncertain.

To bolster the bill's chances of becoming law, some experts propose amalgamating it with more comprehensive cannabis reform legislation like the Marijuana Opportunity Reinvestment and Expungement Act (MORE Act) or the Cannabis Administration and Opportunity Act (CAOA). These broader acts delve into the realm of federal cannabis legalization or decriminalization.

The primary objective of the SAFER Banking Act is to bridge the gap between financial regulations and cannabis laws. This harmony ensures equitable treatment for cannabis-related businesses, which, in turn, promotes a shift away from cash-centric operations. Employees could expect easier access to financial services, from mortgages to formal proof of employment. While the bill enjoys bipartisan support, it also faces opposition from various quarters within both political parties.

How might this legislation impact the cannabis industry? This bill could usher in several favorable changes for the cannabis sector. These potential benefits include:

- *Mitigating Security Risks:* One of the foremost advantages is the reduction of safety hazards associated with cash-only operations. By enabling legal marijuana businesses to access traditional banks, the bill could curtail the vulnerability to theft, fraud, and violent incidents.

- *Enhancing Financial Access:* Access to capital and credit, which has been a formidable challenge for cannabis businesses, could see significant improvement. This would particularly benefit small and minority-owned enterprises, providing them with opportunities for financing that were previously elusive.
- *Transparency and Accountability:* The bill holds the potential to enhance transparency and accountability within the cannabis industry. By permitting financial institutions to monitor, report, and adhere to anti-money laundering regulations, it could foster a more regulated and compliant environment.
- *Industry Growth:* Beyond these advantages, the legislation might catalyze the growth and evolution of the cannabis sector and its related industries, including real estate. It could open doors for increased investment, acquisitions, leasing, and the expansion of cannabis-related properties.

Senator Sherrod Brown of Ohio aptly notes, "Without full access to the banking and payments system, legal cannabis businesses are forced to operate in the shadows." Senator Tim Scott of South Carolina emphasizes Congress's responsibility to ensure that all legal industries have access to financial institutions and services.

Despite the possibilities the Bank Act sets forth, there are several challenges and drawbacks that warrant consideration. For example, the bill does not address the foundational issue of federal cannabis prohibition. This means that cannabis businesses and consumers may still face legal risks and uncertainties despite the legislation. Without proper regulation and enforcement, the bill could inadvertently create opportunities for money laundering and other illicit activities. Furthermore, within the Senate, the bill faces opposition and potential delays. Some lawmakers advocate for a more comprehensive approach to cannabis reform, while others remain staunchly opposed to legalization altogether. These differing viewpoints hinder the bill's progress through the legislative process.

With so much activity, the state legalization map in the US is always changing. Here is the count as of today (February 2024):

- Recreationally Legal: 24 states
- Exclusively Legal for Medical Use: 15 states
- Severely Limited Access: 9 states.

Selling cannabis is not necessarily hard. The demand is there, and the number of people eager to grow, manufacture, and sell the plant is also abundant. However, the most daunting challenge facing cannabis businesses is the exorbitant tax rates we are subject to, courtesy of federal laws that still classify them alongside illegal drug traffickers, as well as excessive city, state, and excise taxation. In addition to this, the prohibition on interstate cannabis commerce forces companies to construct separate facilities, from farms and factories to retail stores, in every state they operate. This requirement not only multiplies their operational expenses but also compels us to adapt to a constantly changing mosaic of state-specific regulations. Furthermore, obtaining the necessary capital for such expansive ventures is notably challenging, given the limited financing options available. This is a pain point acknowledged by both sides of the political aisle in Congress, although no concrete steps have been taken to address it.

That being said, one thing I have learned in my years of experience as a canna-preneur is that in a newly regulated industry like cannabis, every segment is essentially uncharted territory, presenting both challenges and opportunities in equal measure. While navigating this landscape comes with its own set of complications, the potential for innovation and gain is immense. Those who are willing to brave the uncertainties, adapt quickly, and take calculated risks stand to reap substantial rewards as the market matures. So, while the complexities

can be daunting, they also serve as gateways to unparalleled opportunities for those bold enough to seize them.

Cannabis Wall Street: IPOs & RTOs, and Crowdfunding

Cannabis is indeed making its mark on Wall Street. The emerging
industry has attracted considerable interest from investors and entrepreneurs alike, leading to numerous initial public offerings (IPOs),
reverse takeovers (RTOs), and crowdfunding efforts.

The entry of cannabis-related companies into stock markets via
IPOs has been a significant development for an industry with a lack of
capital access challenge. IPOs offer companies the ability to raise
substantial capital for growth while providing investors the opportunity
to participate in the company's potential success.

In the context of the cannabis industry, Marijuana Inc., now known
as Medical Marijuana Inc., was indeed one of the pioneers. Medical
Marijuana Inc. was the first publicly held company vested in the
cannabis and industrial hemp space in North America. It started
trading publicly in 2009, which was a groundbreaking move at that
time considering the legal status of cannabis.

An IPO involves a company creating new shares that it sells to
institutional investors. Depending on demand, these institutional
investors might also sell their holdings to retail investors. The price of
the shares during the IPO is set based on a valuation done by investment banks, which coordinate the IPO process.

However, not all cannabis companies have opted for the traditional
IPO route. Many cannabis companies, for instance, have opted for a
Reverse Takeover (RTO), where a private company acquires a publicly
traded company to bypass the lengthy and complex process of an IPO.
This was the case with some of the biggest names in the industry, such
as Canopy Growth Corporation and Aurora Cannabis.

These IPOs and RTOs have allowed cannabis companies to tap
into larger capital markets and have marked a significant milestone in
the mainstream acknowledgment of the cannabis industry. As legal

restrictions continue to ease up worldwide, we can expect the trend of cannabis companies going public to continue, offering more opportunities for investors and growth for the companies themselves.

Have you ever heard of penny stocks? Well, when it comes to the cannabis industry, there are a number of companies whose shares fall into the penny stock category. These can include smaller growers and retailers, as well as companies providing ancillary services to the cannabis industry, such as hydroponics suppliers, consulting services, or cannabis-related biotech firms.

Please be advised that investing in cannabis penny stocks carries the same risks as investing in any other penny stock. In addition to the normal risks associated with small-cap stocks, the cannabis industry faces additional uncertainties. As we discussed in prior chapters, this includes the ever-changing regulatory environment surrounding the plant, especially in the United States, where, as of today (May 2024), federal and state laws can be at odds.

Despite these risks, some investors are drawn to cannabis penny stocks because of the potential for high returns. The global legal cannabis market is expected to grow significantly in the coming years, and if smaller cannabis firms can establish a strong position in the market, they could potentially provide substantial returns in the near future. When considering investing in cannabis or any penny stocks, it's important to do thorough research and understand that these investments can be highly risky. You should only invest money that you can afford to lose, and it may be wise to seek advice from a financial adviser before making these types of investments.

An interesting development in the industry has been the use of Regulation A offerings, which are a type of offering that allows private companies to raise up to $75 million from both accredited and non-accredited investors. *High Times*, the historically well-known cannabis-related publication turned plant-touching operator we mentioned in an earlier chapter, utilized Regulation A for their offering, allowing everyday cannabis enthusiasts and supporters to become shareholders.

Gage Cannabis, a cannabis brand and operator in Michigan, also used a Regulation A offering to raise capital. This approach offers an innovative way for smaller investors to participate in the financial development of companies they support.

Prime Harvest Inc., the company for which I serve as Chief Marketing Officer, also received a qualification from the US Securities and Exchange Commission to raise capital under Regulation A. Weed4ThePeople.com is your chance to own a part of Prime Harvest Inc. and your opportunity to help create a new benchmark in safe cannabis access and investment for all through the expansion of Jaxx Cannabis, our flagship store, and delivery platform. Weed 4 the People is our awareness campaign to attract like-minded investors to participate in our business as shareholders. For more information, please check out www.weed4thepeople.com.

Overall, these financial developments reflect a larger trend of growing acceptance of the cannabis industry. As laws and attitudes continue to evolve, the industry's financial landscape will likely continue to grow and diversify, creating new opportunities for both businesses and investors alike.

The Age of Technology

In nearly a decade of experience in the cannabis industry, I've witnessed firsthand how technology is revolutionizing every aspect of the business. Canna-tech is not just an emerging field; it's a transformative force that's reshaping how cannabis is cultivated, sold, and experienced by consumers. It's also streamlining operations across the entire supply chain, from cultivation and processing to distribution, marketing, and consumption. This vibrant intersection of technology and cannabis is filled with exciting new possibilities, and it's setting the stage for unprecedented innovation.

The application of technology within the cannabis industry has evolved into a powerful tool for tackling a range of industry-specific challenges. From meeting stringent regulatory guidelines to ensuring product quality and consistency, technology is at the forefront of the sector's innovation. Moreover, tech-driven solutions are enhancing customer education and extending market reach, acting as a catalyst for sustainable growth and development in the industry.

Cannabis cultivation, traditionally an artisanal, small-scale operation, is now becoming increasingly industrialized and sophisticated. The proliferation of advanced technologies such as automated growing systems, specialized LED lighting solutions, and plant tissue culture techniques are significantly augmenting the cultivation process. These technologies not only maximize efficiency and yield but also ensure a consistent, high-quality product, which is paramount in the medicinal cannabis vertical.

Even government regulatory entities rely on technology to implement track and trace systems like Metrc to manage comprehensive seed-to-sale tracking. Their goal is to ensure product safety and to mitigate the risk of illegal diversion. I must say, these types of programs are a work in progress.

Earlier, I mentioned Weedmaps and Leafly. Online platforms in the form of native apps and Web2 like them are quintessential examples of technology bridging the gap between cannabis businesses and consumers. They offer information on cannabis strains, products, and dispensaries while serving as a marketing tool for businesses looking to target a wider range of customers.

The retail aspect of the cannabis industry has also been revolutionized by the advent of sophisticated point-of-sale (POS) systems, e-commerce platforms, and delivery apps, all tailor-made for the cannabis market. These technological tools assist in managing inventory, optimizing sales, ensuring regulatory compliance, and offering valuable business insights.

The potential of emerging technologies like web3, the metaverse, and artificial intelligence in the cannabis industry is also starting to be recognized. These technologies could offer new avenues for consumer education, immersive marketing experiences, remote social events, predictive market analytics, and possibly more efficient money management. Don't forget to check out BSW Nation in the Spatial.io metaverse. BSW Nation presents an immersive experience of a few advocacy campaigns by the lifestyle brand Boycott Shitty Weed.

40 Tons, a social impact cannabis company, also uses web3 technologies to promote the mission of their brand. The company's goal is to help free the over 40,000 prisoners still imprisoned over nonviolent cannabis offenses in the United States. The 40 Tons team aims to use technology as a resource to achieve this impressive deed through their NFT Project, *40 Tons of NFTs*.

Technology in the cannabis industry acts as a powerful catalyst for innovation, problem-solving, and growth. Whether it's software for compliance and inventory management, hardware for precise cultivation conditions, or advanced extraction techniques, technology is reshaping the landscape of how we do business. From my early days at Prime Harvest Inc., it was clear that we were not just a cannabis organization but a technology-driven one. My initiation into this tech-centric ethos began with conversations with Duane, my business partner who is also an unabashed plant nerd. Duane always emphasized the transformative potential of plant tissue culture technology for the cannabis sector. With his guidance, I came to realize this technology has the power to revolutionize quality control, scalability, and sustainability in our field. The implementation of this technology lets us generate plants that are genetic clones of a parent, ensuring that each plant possesses the exact same cannabinoid and terpene profiles. This uniformity is indispensable, especially when it comes to medical cannabis, where consistent potency and dosing are paramount.

Tissue culture's ability to produce many plants in a compact area not only makes it a cost-efficient technique but also a sustainable one. By reducing the square footage needed for cultivation, we are simultaneously shrinking our environmental footprint, a crucial move for an industry that aims to be responsible and sustainable. Equally important, the sterile environment of tissue culture minimizes the threat of pests and diseases, reducing our reliance on pesticides and aligning us better with stringent regulatory requirements for product safety.

For me, the prospect of a uniform and reliable cannabis market isn't just a pipe dream; it's an achievable reality on the near horizon. Imagine the simple yet profound joy of finding your favorite strain from a trusted brand in California and then walking into a dispensary in NYC and finding that exact same product. The potential of plant tissue culture to make this a reality is tantalizing. As a committed cannapreneur with a long-term vision, the quest to solve such grand challenges is both my midnight muse and my morning motivation. It keeps me up, but it also propels me forward to keep on keeping on in this complex yet amazing industry.

While technology has already brought about significant changes to the industry, we are just at the beginning of this exciting journey. As the space continues to expand and the legal landscape becomes more conducive, the role of technology in shaping the future of cannabis is set to become even more profound. The integration of technology and cannabis is poised to push the boundaries of innovation, creating a safer and more efficient cannabis industry.

Community Impact

From the grassroots activists who rallied for medical cannabis legislation to the burgeoning online forums that act as a treasure trove of user experiences and advice, cannabis communities have always been the lifeblood of this industry. Their role isn't merely peripheral; it's foundational. These communities serve as the crucible for ideas, policy initiatives, and education, becoming an essential hallmark that informs the sector's direction at large.

The vibrancy of these communities is drawn from their diversity. They range from veterans who seek solace in cannabis for symptoms of PTSD to women who are breaking glass ceilings in cannabis entrepreneurship. There are communities of moms advocating for CBD as an alternative for children with epilepsy and trade communities that help standardize commercial practices. The LGBTQ+ community has also been a staunch advocate for both medical and recreational use, adding another layer of rich dialogue to the conversation.

In this industry, there is always a focus on wellness, with communities discussing cannabis as part of a holistic lifestyle beyond mere recreational or medicinal use. From infused yoga classes to meditation sessions accompanied by doses of THC, cannabis has found its way into diverse wellness routines. And let's not forget the invaluable input from medical patients, who share firsthand experiences and thereby shape the kinds of products that end up on the shelves. They serve as real-world testers, helping to fine-tune everything from dosage to delivery methods.

In a world that's increasingly digital, these communities also thrive online, facilitating a global exchange of ideas and practices that transcends borders. Whether it's an online forum for growers, a subreddit for cannabis recipes, or a Twitter thread debating the latest legislation, these platforms foster a collective intelligence, pooling knowledge that any interested party can tap into.

So, as we navigate the complexity and uniqueness of the cannabis landscape, these communities act as our North Star, continually offering insights, validation, or challenges to the prevailing norms. Their collective voice doesn't just echo in empty chambers; it resonates in legislative halls, impacts commercial strategies, and shapes public perception. Cannabis communities are not just observers or consumers; they are active co-creators of the cannabis narrative, and their significance cannot be overstated.

Veteran groups such as Veterans Walk and Talk (VWAT) serve as strong advocates for the use of plant medicine in managing PTSD, pain management, and other conditions prevalent in the veteran community. The non-profit organization is a critical voice in the discussions centered around safe access to cannabis and other natural therapies for military veterans and their families, especially for those seeking alternatives to traditional pharmaceutical treatments.

The primary objective of VWAT is to equip veterans with the tools and resources necessary to independently manage their health. VWAT utilizes a multifaceted approach incorporating physical exercise, cannabis, psychedelics, and a supportive community. Engaging in introspection within a secure environment has been shown to alleviate numerous challenges faced by veterans and their families. By combining "walk and talk" therapy with various wellness modalities, VWAT has created an effective formula for veterans to engage in personal growth and healing.

Another great veteran organization is the Veteran Action Council. The Veteran Action Council is a dedicated collective of military veterans and professionals from various fields who come together in a volunteer capacity to advocate for and organize initiatives centered on enabling veterans access to alternative treatments and therapies. By doing so, they aspire to enhance the physical and mental well-being of both veterans and their families.

Their shared commitment and efforts have resulted in the creation and submission of a "Green Paper" to the White House ONDCP. This significant action was a response to the ONDCP's call for public insight into its policies, particularly those that may have negative implications for certain sections of society. Through their continual advocacy and active participation, the Veteran Action Council strives to contribute to making meaningful changes that uplift the health and well-being of the veteran community.

Women-led communities like The Pink Sesh, Blunt Brunch, Latinas in Cannabis, and Supernova Women bring a much-needed female perspective to an industry that has historically been male-dominated. These groups foster a sense of empowerment and inclusivity, advocating for female representation in the cannabis industry. They offer spaces for women to learn, network, and share their experiences with cannabis, contributing to a shift in the perception and understanding of the plant.

BIPOC communities, such as Minorities for Medical Marijuana, play an indispensable role in the fight for equity in the cannabis industry. They work tirelessly to combat the disproportionate effects of cannabis prohibition on communities of color while advocating for diverse representation and equal opportunities within the industry.

The Indigenous Cannabis Industry Association (ICIA) is playing a crucial role in supporting the 574 federally recognized American Indian tribes as they explore the cannabis industry. By promoting cannabis education and development that directly benefits tribal communities, the ICIA aims to foster economic growth and healthcare advancements within these often-marginalized groups. Additionally, the organization acts as a unifying network, helping tribes navigate the complicated patchwork of state-by-state cannabis regulations.

The LGBTQ+ community, long intertwined with cannabis advocacy due to the HIV/AIDS crisis, continues to be a strong advocate for legalization and equal access. They highlight the importance of inclusive spaces within the cannabis world and push for acknowledgment and respect for all users. This is Jane Project is a non-profit organization that sheds light, builds community, and uplifts the lives of women and nonbinary trauma survivors. The program's trauma-aware curriculum is designed to support the organization's mission through community building, healing services, and compassionate care facilitation (donated medicine).

Medical patients comprise an indispensable part of the cannabis community. Their experiences, stories, and advocacy efforts have significantly contributed to the shifting perspectives around cannabis and have been instrumental in advancing its acceptance and legalization.

Patients who use cannabis for medicinal purposes form a diverse group, encompassing people of all ages and backgrounds who suffer from a wide variety of health conditions. From those managing chronic pain, epilepsy, multiple sclerosis, and glaucoma to individuals utilizing cannabis as an adjunct therapy in cancer treatment or as a means to alleviate symptoms of mental health disorders such as PTSD and anxiety, these individuals are at the forefront of demonstrating the therapeutic potential of cannabis.

These patients' personal experiences often stand as powerful testimonials to the efficacy of cannabis, offering hope to others dealing with similar health issues. Through their shared experiences, a strong community has formed. The medical patient community has not only provided a supportive network for individuals navigating their medical journeys but also has become a persuasive force advocating for further research, understanding, and acceptance of cannabis as a legitimate therapeutic option.

Patient advocacy groups and organizations play a pivotal role in this landscape. They work tirelessly to challenge the stigma associated with cannabis use, lobby for legal changes that improve patient access, and provide education about the potential benefits and risks of cannabis therapy. Their work directly impacts policy, healthcare practices, and societal attitudes toward medicinal cannabis.

Medical patients, therefore, are not merely passive recipients in the cannabis narrative. They are active contributors, shaping the course of the cannabis industry through their personal experiences, collective voice, and persistent advocacy. They embody the human aspect of the cannabis dialogue, reminding us that, at its core, the drive toward cannabis legalization and normalization is about improving quality of life and advocating for patient choice in healthcare.

The impact of these communities cannot be overstated. They are the beating heart of the cannabis movement, driving it forward, infusing it with diversity, and ensuring it stays true to its roots in compassion, advocacy, and social justice. Their voices amplify the message that cannabis is not only a product but a plant with the power to heal, connect, and transform society.

Cannabis has been used by humans for thousands of years, and as such, it has a rich history of exploration, study, and research. The story of cannabis research is a compelling one, tracing from ancient civilizations' usage and understanding to the contemporary era's scientific discoveries and advancements.

As stated in earlier chapters, ancient societies recognized cannabis for its potential medicinal or psychoactive properties. Throughout the ages, the properties of cannabis were described in various ancient texts. In ancient China, around 2700 BC, Emperor Shen Nung, considered the father of Chinese medicine, wrote about cannabis in his pharmacopoeia, referring to its medicinal properties. Similarly, in India, cannabis has been a part of religious and cultural rituals and has also been utilized in Ayurvedic medicine for centuries.

The journey of cannabis research took a significant turn in the nineteenth century when Western medicine began to take an interest in the plant. In the 1840s, Irish physician William O'Shaughnessy, who worked in India, conducted some of the first clinical trials on cannabis, reporting its potential as an analgesic and muscle relaxant. However, it wasn't until the twentieth century when scientific research began to truly unlock the potential of cannabis. The key breakthrough came in 1964, when Israeli scientists Raphael Mechoulam and Yechiel Gaoni identified and synthesized Delta-9-tetrahydrocannabinol (THC), the primary psychoactive compound in cannabis.

The subsequent decades saw a surge of interest and research, leading to the discovery of the endocannabinoid system in the human body in the 1990s, a complex network of receptors and compounds that interact with cannabinoids and are believed to play a crucial role in maintaining the body's homeostasis.

Despite legal and societal restrictions, the twenty-first century has seen an explosion of research into cannabis, with studies exploring its potential therapeutic benefits for a host of conditions including epilepsy, multiple sclerosis, chronic pain, and more.

In 2018, I had the incredible opportunity to collaborate with Dr. Cristina Sanchez, a leading figure in cannabinoid research, particularly its applications in cancer treatment. She was one of our esteemed speakers at the second Cannabis 4 The Cause educational event in San Diego. Dr. Sanchez traveled all the way from Spain to shed light on her groundbreaking research, offering valuable insights into the complex relationship between cannabinoids and cancer cells reduction.

Dr. Sanchez's journey in cannabinoid research began in her undergraduate years at Universidad Complutense of Madrid, where she initially explored the impact of cannabinoids on lipid and carbohydrate intermediate metabolism. After completing her PhD in Biochemistry and Molecular Biology, she delved deeper into her research focus: examining the effects of cannabinoids on cancer cell proliferation. Her postdoctoral work in California under a doctor named Piomelli expanded her expertise to include other bioactive lipids and their roles in pain initiation.

Returning to Spain with a coveted "Ramón y Cajal" contract, a program designed to bring Spanish researchers back to their homeland, Dr. Sanchez coordinated a new research line in collaboration with a local lab. Her primary goal is to decode the intricate role of the endocannabinoid system in breast cancer. Her work aims not only to identify new therapeutic targets but also to provide more refined screening tools with both prognostic and predictive values for breast cancer patients.

Aside from her lab work, Dr. Sanchez holds prominent positions in several Spanish scientific organizations. She serves as the Vice President of the Spanish Cannabinoid Research Society, is the Secretary and a founding member of the Spanish Observatory on Medical Cannabis, and the Vice Dean of Research at the School of Biology at Complutense University.

It's rare to find someone with such comprehensive expertise in this niche yet incredibly important field. Dr. Sanchez's commitment to her research and her eagerness to share her knowledge contributes significantly to the cannabis community, academia, and most importantly, to the lives of countless patients who may benefit from cannabinoid-based treatments in the future.

Historically, cannabis research in the United States has been heavily restricted due to its Schedule I status under the Controlled Substances Act, which categorizes it as a drug with high potential for abuse and no accepted medical use. This status has made it difficult for researchers to obtain cannabis for study and has limited the funding available for such research.

However, there have been ongoing discussions and efforts in Congress to ease these restrictions and improve access to cannabis for research purposes:

Medical Marijuana Research Act

In a major federal policy shift, President Biden signed into law the "Medical Marijuana and Cannabidiol Research Expansion Act, H.R. 8454," (commonly known as the Cannabis Research Bill) on December 2, 2022. A product of bipartisan consensus, this legislation is the first stand-alone cannabis reform bill to gain approval from both the House and Senate, marking a crucial turning point in the history of federal cannabis policy.

While the new law does not alter cannabis's Schedule I classification, its intent is manifold: to promote research into the potential risks and medical benefits of cannabis and cannabis products, streamline the DEA's role in this research, expand sources of research-grade cannabis, facilitate the commercial development of FDA-approved drugs derived from cannabis and hemp, and to ensure that physicians can freely discuss the potential risks and benefits of cannabis with their patients. Being able to fund and carry out research without federal penalties places us closer to being able to further unlock the potential of cannabis.

The Cannabis Research Bill was proposed in July 2022 by Representatives Earl Blumenauer (D-OR) and Andy Harris, MD (R-MD), among others. After swift passage in the House, the Senate gave its approval in a voice vote on November 16, 2022. The bill resolved long-standing differences between research expansion proposals passed by the House and the Senate in the 117th Congress (2021-2022).

Previously, clinical research involving cannabis had to navigate a multi-step process involving three federal agencies: the FDA, the DEA, and the NIDA. Additionally, they had to adhere to the requirements set forth by the states in which the research was conducted. These federal procedures governed scientific research protocols as security measures to prevent diversion and control the source of the cannabis used in the research.

Now, under the new legislation, DEA's process for registering cannabis research applicants is streamlined, with specific timelines for review of applications and adjustments in study protocols. Furthermore, the bill ensures an adequate and uninterrupted supply of cannabis for research purposes, a significant improvement over previous restrictions that left many researchers displeased with the lack of diversity and supply of products available for study.

Another important aspect of the bill is the provision of a safe harbor for institutions of higher education. These institutions had long been concerned that conducting cannabis research could jeopardize their federal funding due to prohibitions in the Drug-Free Schools and Campuses Act (DFSCA) of cannabis possession, use, or distribution.

Moreover, the bill also offers a measure of clarity for potential investors in clinical research involving the plant. It mandates DEA to register applicants seeking to manufacture or distribute cannabis for the commercial production of FDA-approved cannabis-derived products. Title III of the bill expressly allows physicians to discuss with their patients the potential risks and benefits of cannabis derivatives and CBD as treatments. This exemption is particularly significant for veterans, who have been advocating for cannabis to be considered as a treatment for post-traumatic stress disorder, chronic pain, and other disabling conditions.

Last, the bill mandates a report to Congress on Federal Research, requiring HHS to submit a report on the therapeutic potential of cannabis or CBD for serious medical conditions, including intractable epilepsy, and the potential impact of increasing THC levels on the human body and developing adolescent brains. We hope that this legislation is a stride toward enabling more research and understanding of the potential therapeutic benefits and risks of cannabis and its derivatives.

The study of cannabis has indeed come a long way from the time of Shen Nung, who's alleged work, the "Shen Nong Ben Cao Jing," is one of the earliest pharmacopoeias. However, the complexity of the plant, with its hundreds of cannabinoids, and the legal challenges faced by researchers, means that there is still much to be explored and understood. As attitudes and laws around cannabis continue to evolve, we can anticipate a future where the full potential of this ancient plant is realized through rigorous scientific research.

Justice System Concerns

Not the cannabis plant causing a burden on the justice system! The influence of cannabis on the American and global justice system is a convoluted subject that touches on many social, legal, and ethical issues. It would be too easy and lazy to say cannabis is the blame for this or that. But the reality is that the unwarranted policies set forth by politicians and systemic racism is really the guilty party in this case. In the United States, cannabis has been at the forefront of political and legal debates for decades, with the "War on Drugs" policy exacerbating social inequalities, mass incarceration, and systemic disenfranchisement of vulnerable communities. Its effects ripple beyond national boundaries, affecting drug policies and justice systems worldwide.

The War on Drugs launched in the 1970s to combat drug use and trafficking through stringent criminalization laws. Rather than curbing drug addiction and trafficking, it led to the mass incarceration of individuals, primarily for cannabis and other nonviolent drug offenses. Disproportionately impacted were minority communities, particularly African Americans and Hispanics/Latin communities, who found themselves the targets of selective law enforcement actions. The racial disparities in cannabis-related arrests are staggering; Black Americans are nearly four times as likely to be arrested for cannabis possession as their white counterparts, despite similar rates of use among both groups.

The criminalization of cannabis has broad societal ramifications beyond the staggering rates of imprisonment. Convictions lead to long-lasting consequences like employment restrictions, loss of voting rights, and diminished educational opportunities. These outcomes collectively contribute to a cycle of poverty and disenfranchisement, perpetuating systemic inequality. This effect is most pronounced in vulnerable communities already facing socioeconomic challenges, essentially criminalizing poverty and minority status.

The toll on criminal justice resources is also significant. Law enforcement agencies devote enormous manpower and financial resources to cannabis-related arrests and prosecutions, often at the expense of more serious crimes. In states where cannabis is still illegal, police officers spend countless hours pursuing, arresting, and processing individuals for low-level cannabis offenses. These efforts strain judicial and penal systems, crowding courts and prisons and leaving less room and attention for violent and high-impact crimes.

The effects on border states, particularly those sharing boundaries with states where cannabis is legal, add another layer of complexity. Inconsistencies in state laws have given rise to a complicated patchwork of regulations, making it challenging for law enforcement agencies to enforce laws efficiently and fairly. The disparities in cannabis laws between states also encourage a form of "drug tourism," where individuals travel to states with legalized cannabis to make a purchase, then return to their home state where possession may be illegal, thus exposing themselves to criminal liability.

Globally, the American stance on cannabis has had a considerable influence. US foreign policy, historically funding and supporting international drug control programs, has often prioritized cannabis criminalization. Countries receiving American aid frequently model their drug laws after US policies, perpetuating issues like mass incarceration, systemic discrimination, and prevention of access to medical patients. However, a seemingly about-face in American public opinion and legislative reforms are slowly diverging global perspectives toward a more openminded direction. Countries like Colombia, a few African countries, and several European nations are reevaluating their cannabis laws, some opting for decriminalization or outright legalization.

In recent years, some American states have taken steps to redress the wrongs of the past by legalizing cannabis, expunging prior convictions, and creating social equity programs within their cannabis regulations. However, these reforms vary widely from state to state and don't fully address the systemic issues created by decades of cannabis criminalization. While state-level reforms provide a starting point, comprehensive federal action is necessary to address the far-reaching impacts of cannabis on the American and global justice system.

The influence of cannabis on the justice system is profound and widespread, affecting not just those who consume, sell, grow or produce the plant and derived products but also society at large. It challenges the ethical foundations of criminal justice, disproportionately affects minority communities, and drains vital resources that could be better spent on addressing more severe crimes. As attitudes toward cannabis evolve, there is a growing need for a comprehensive and unified approach to its legal status. One that accounts for its complex history, its impact on vulnerable populations, the prioritization of access to patients and adults, its role in the global landscape, and its sustainability implications.

In recent years, our understanding of the endocannabinoid system (ECS) and its intricate relationship with cannabis has blossomed. The ECS, named after its interaction with cannabis, plays a vital role in our bodies, extending far beyond the world of cannabinoids.

Imagine a complex system within your body that continuously strives to maintain optimal stability regardless of external influences. This state, known as homeostasis, is like the gauges on an airplane dashboard—they alert the operator about deviations from ideal conditions. Much like these instruments, your body constantly monitors critical levels and functions, such as temperature, hormone balance, heart rate, hunger, and waste accumulation. When something falls outside the optimal range, the ECS steps in to correct it. For instance, when you're overheated and begin to sweat, thank your ECS for helping cool you down. If your mouth is dry, it's a reminder from your ECS that you need to hydrate.

This remarkable system involves three key components:

- *Endocannabinoids*: These are the natural compounds our bodies produce.

- *Receptors:* Found throughout the nervous system and various body tissues, these receptors interact with both endocannabinoids and external cannabinoids.
- *Enzymes:* These play a crucial role in breaking down endocannabinoids and cannabinoids.

Beyond just being a natural part of our biology, the ECS is fundamental. You've likely heard numerous claims about the medicinal potential of cannabis. While it may seem like hype, medical science increasingly supports many of these assertions. The wide-ranging effects stem from the expansive reach of the ECS.

To understand this fully, let's explore in further detail the role of receptors and enzymes within the ECS. According to health.harvard.edu, when an individual smokes cannabis, the cannabinoid known as THC binds to CB1 receptors in the brain, resulting in a euphoric feeling. This is where the term "delta-9-tetrahydrocannabinol" (THC) comes from. Remarkably, your body produces an endocannabinoid called anandamide that also binds to CB1 receptors, but it doesn't induce a high. Instead, anandamide has a calming effect.

The enzyme FAAH plays a pivotal role in this distinction. It swiftly breaks down endocannabinoids created by your body, like anandamide, but it cannot metabolize THC. Consequently, THC lingers longer in the system, leading to more pronounced effects.

Cannabidiol (known as CBD), another plant-based cannabinoid, has garnered significant attention from researchers. Unlike THC, it lacks psychoactive properties, offering the benefits of cannabis without the "high." CBD appears to prevent FAAH from breaking down anandamide effectively, allowing it to have a more profound impact. This property explains why CBD is explored as a treatment for anxiety disorders.

Medical science has uncovered conditions associated with ECS dysregulation, collectively termed clinical endocannabinoid deficiency (CECD). CECD isn't a disease itself but encompasses conditions sharing this common feature.

Conditions with potential links to CECD include fibromyalgia, migraine, and irritable bowel syndrome. These conditions often resist conventional treatments, prompting research into cannabis-based remedies.

These disorders typically affect multiple systems, reflecting the widespread influence of the ECS. For example, fibromyalgia involves the central and peripheral nervous systems, the immune system, hormonal balance, and digestive function. It has also been linked to issues like premature perimenopause, conception difficulties, and early hysterectomy, alongside symptoms like temperature sensitivity and memory problems.

Though the exact mechanisms remain unclear, the ECS appears integral to maintaining homeostasis, and its dysregulation can manifest as these complex disorders. Research into rectifying endocannabinoid deficiency is ongoing, with cannabis and hemp products gaining acceptance within patient communities.

Cannabinoids are currently under intensive research for their potential to treat various conditions, extending beyond endocannabinoid deficiency-related disorders. Researchers are exploring their potential in treating Alzheimer's, cardiovascular disease, neurological and psychiatric illnesses, kidney disease, autoimmune diseases, chronic inflammatory conditions, and chronic pain.

CBD, specifically, is already utilized for pediatric epilepsy, pain management, inflammation control, acne treatment, asthma relief, and more. The National Institutes of Health's National Center for Complementary and Integrative Health notes that cannabis has been employed in medical treatment for over 3,000 years, addressing an array of conditions like pain, digestive issues, and psychological disorders. Earlier chapters illustrate such a timeline. While debates over the safety and efficacy of cannabis persist, it is predominantly used for pain relief, eating disorders, nausea, glaucoma, anxiety, and seizures in the United States and other parts of the world.

The opioid epidemic has propelled interest in alternative analgesics, with over 62% of medical cannabis users citing chronic pain relief as their primary reason for consumption. Additionally, an intriguing study published in the Journal of Health Economics (July 2023) has revealed a connection between adult-use cannabis laws and reduced tobacco use. This is particularly significant, as the normalization of cannabis through legalization was feared to undermine tobacco control policies.

The study highlights three key findings:

- Adult-use cannabis laws led to a 2%–5% increase in prior-month cannabis use, including vaping, primarily among individuals who had not previously consumed cannabis.
- There is no evidence that adult-use cannabis laws increased adult tobacco use. Instead, these laws were associated with a gradual decline in all forms of tobacco use, including cigarettes, pipe tobacco, cigars, electronic cigarettes, and nicotine vaporizers, after two to three years of their enactment.
- The availability of dispensaries played a pivotal role in reducing tobacco use, with states that allowed dispensaries experiencing up to a 2% reduction in tobacco use after two to three years of legalization.

This study's findings offer valuable insights into the impact of cannabis legalization on public health. Longitudinal data enable a more comprehensive analysis of tobacco use trends over time, enhancing our understanding of the relationship between cannabis laws and tobacco. With time and proper documentation, data gathered will paint a more complete picture.

Chapter 12
The Green Renaissance Awaits

I named this book *Green Renaissance*, not as a cannabis buzzword but as a tribute to the cultural, scientific, and economic rebirth that's revolutionizing our society from the ground up. So, what roles do we play as individuals, communities, and nations in this transformative era?

The renaissance is here; the future is now. As we discussed in the previous chapters, individuals, communities, and governments play essential roles in this unfolding generational shift. From individual choices about consumption to collective advocacy for policy reform, every action contributes to the future of our planet. A future that includes the cannabis plant as a valuable resource. And so, as we leap forward, the question becomes not just what the future holds for this growing industry but how each of us can be active participants in shaping that future today.

The green renaissance signals a paradigm shift in how we perceive and interact with the plant. It's not just about CBD oils lining the shelves of health stores or cannabis-themed cafés popping up in cities; it's a reimagining of an entire industry and its place in our communities as part of our wellness, lifestyle, and culture. This development is not confined to just the limits of the cannabis industry but extends to our broader social fabric, influencing individual behaviors, community norms, business practices, and government policies.

Every individual has the power to contribute and, in many ways, influence this green renaissance. Each choice we make about cannabis, whether it's deciding to use it for medicinal purposes, supporting a local cannabis business, or simply engaging in dialogue to discuss and dispel long-standing stigmas, carries a significant impact. History shows, time and time again, that our individual actions, in aggregate, have the power to change societal attitudes, encourage scientific exploration, and facilitate a more nuanced understanding and curiosity about all subjects, cannabis included.

One thing that has remained consistent within this ever-changing space is the fact that community is the backbone shaping the trajectory of this movement. Grassroots advocacy has been the bedrock of cannabis reform, with communities coming together to push for policy changes, educate the public, and provide support for those affected by cannabis prohibition. Local initiatives, such as those advocating for safe access, social equity, and social justice reform in cannabis, are vital in ensuring that the benefits of the industry are shared equitably.

On a broader level, the role of governments in enabling and shaping the green renaissance cannot be overstated. Decisions made at the legislative and regulatory levels determine the robustness of the legal landscape in which the cannabis industry operates. With that being said, policymakers have a responsibility to enact laws that reflect evolving public attitudes toward cannabis, protect consumers, promote equity, and facilitate economic growth. Advocacy for sensible, just, and forward-thinking policies is a crucial component for the full economic integration of cannabis in society.

As we stand on the precipice of this transformative time period, we have an opportunity to not just be passive observers waiting to see what the future holds. Instead, we can be active participants, with the power to shape the future of a revitalized and exciting cannabis space. Whether it's through normalization efforts, education, community advocacy, or pushing for policy reform, each of us has a role to play in advancing the future of cannabis.

Looking ahead, the potential of the cannabis industry is vast. From advancements in medicinal cannabis to the growth of a sustainable hemp industry, the opportunities are boundless. But this future is not guaranteed. It relies on our continued efforts to advocate for change, challenge outdated perceptions, and ensure that the green revolution realizes its full potential. So, as we peer into this exciting path, let's also reflect on the power we hold in the present. The future of cannabis is indeed now, and it's in the palm of our hands.

Why I Wrote This Book

With this book, I set out to share a vision that has fueled my passion and defined my life's work: a vision of a future where cannabis is not just decriminalized but seamlessly integrated into every facet of our societies in which the plant can add value. It is a future where cannabis, revered as a potent plant medicine, has its healing potential entirely harnessed for health and wellness. It's a world where the socioeconomic benefits of the cannabis industry are far-reaching, contributing to the prosperity of communities worldwide. It's a world where cannabis not only thrives in our agriculture but underpins our drive for sustainable practices, becoming an integral part of our efforts to live more harmoniously with the environment.

The genesis of this book lies deep in my firm conviction about the potential of the cannabis plant. This conviction is shaped by personal experiences and almost a decade of intentional and comprehensive exploration. The cannabis plant has been more than just an area of interest to me; it has been a lifeline. It is the plant that saved my life when I was a young US Navy veteran dealing with PTSD and the ramifications of a traumatic brain injury that took place while on deployment. This intimate connection has amplified my belief in its transformative potential. This book is a product of that belief and a testament to the extraordinary capabilities of cannabis.

Nevertheless, this book is more than a recount of the history of the cannabis plant throughout the ages or my personal optimistic vision of the future of this dynamic industry. It is about the shared journey we are all participating in, whether consciously or unconsciously, as our society shifts its stance on cannabis. It's about examining the past, assessing the present, and contemplating the future of our society and how this exceptional plant can be a vital supporting block within it. It is about fostering a broader dialogue, inspiring reflection, and promoting change in the way we perceive and interact with the plant. And, of course, it is also about giving props to the plant for playing a major role in many aspects of our social construct through the ages.

Green Renaissance was born out of my desire to contribute further to this dialogue, to provide insight, to awaken curiosity, and to provide a foundation of understanding for those intrigued or perplexed by the cannabis plant and its place in our world. It is for the advocates championing change, for the skeptics in need of "more information," for patients seeking alternative therapies, for entrepreneurs eyeing the budding opportunity, and for anyone and everyone eager to comprehend the multifaceted influence of cannabis on our wellness, lifestyle, and culture worldwide.

Most importantly, let it be known that this book is not the end of the journey. It is but a step on the path. The rapidly evolving landscape of cannabis demands constant engagement and continual learning. The discourse on cannabis, its uses, its implications, and its potential is one that invites questions, provokes thought, and challenges preconceived notions.

Now that you have more insight into cannabis, I urge you to keep exploring, to keep asking questions, to keep adding value, and to continue challenging the status quo. We each have a role to play in this unfolding narrative. So, as you navigate this path, consider your role in this green renaissance. What will it look like? How will you influence the future of cannabis?

Personally, the future of cannabis, as I envision it, is not some distant utopia. It is within our grasp. Realizing this vision depends on all of us, on our actions, our advocacy, our activism, and our willingness to embrace the change that is already underway. As you wrap up reading this book, I hope you found not only insight but awaken curiosity. Curiosity to ask more questions to better understand the work of the countless advocates, researchers, patients, entrepreneurs, and consumers propelling this industry forward.

The future we are striving for is one where the value of cannabis is fully acknowledged and its legacy rewritten. This future is not just a dream; it is an imminent reality. So, as we stand at this critical juncture, let's not just be spectators to the green renaissance. Let's be architects.

Bibliography

Dhaval Dave, Yang Liang, Michael F. Pesko, Serena Phillips, Joseph J. Sabia, "Have recreational marijuana laws undermined public health progress on adult tobacco use?", Journal of Health Economics, Volume 90, 2023, 102756, ISSN 0167-6296, https://doi.org/10.1016/j.jhealeco.2023.102756.

Ricardo E. Carrión, Andrea M. Auther, Danielle McLaughlin, Steven Adelsheim, Cynthia Z

Burton, Cameron S Carter, Tara Niendam, J. Daniel Ragland, Tamara G Sale, Stephan F Taylor, Ivy F Tso, William R McFarlane, Barbara A. Cornblatt, "Recreational cannabis use over time in individuals at clinical high risk for psychosis: Lack of associations with symptom, neurocognitive, functioning, and treatment patterns", Psychiatry Research, Volume 328, 2023, 115420, ISSN 0165-1781, https://doi.org/10.1016/j.psychres.2023.115420.

Marijuana on My Mind: The Science and Mystique of Cannabis, pp. 80 – 99. DOI: https://doi.org/10.1017/9781009024983.007 Publisher: Cambridge University Press Print publication year: 2022

"SAFE Banking Act 2023-2024 and Its Impact on the Cannabis Industry." 2024. Cover Cannabis. January 29, 2024. https://covercannabis.com/blog/safe-banking-act-cannabis/.

"Anxiety and Cannabis: A Review of Recent Research." 2023. Medical Cannabis Research Center. April 10, 2023. https://drexel.edu/cannabis-research/research/research-highlights/2023/April/anxiety_cannabis_fact_sheet/.

"News Release." n.d. Feeds.issuerdirect.com. Accessed Novem 19, 2023. https://feeds.issuerdirect.com/news-release.html?newsid=5415833084958573.

"Entheogenic Use of Cannabis." 2020. Wikipedia. June 26, 2020. https://en.wikipedia.org/wiki/Entheogenic_use_of_cannabis.

"Jungmaven Hemp Clothing Review (2023) | the Quality Edit." n.d. Www.thequalityedit.com. Accessed April 27, 2024. https://www.thequalityedit.com/articles/jungmaven-hemp-tshirt-review.

"How Cannabis Is Changing the Way We Dress." n.d. Herb.co. Accessed April 27, 2023. https://herb.co/learn/how-cannabis-is-changing-the-way-we-dress.

Warren, Liz, and Liz Warren. 2021. "Levi's Targets More Hemp, Sustainable Cotton in Jeans." Sourcing Journal. September 27, 2021. https://sourcingjournal.com/denim/denim-brands/levis-cottonized-hemp-organic-cotton-sustainability-report-fiber-innovations-302998/.

"The 420 Code" 2024. The420code.com. 2024. https://the420code.com.

Decarlo, Samantha, and Marin Weaver. 2022. "International Trade Commission Executive Briefings on Trade." https://www.usitc.gov/publications/332/working_papers/ebot_decarlo_weaver_grassroots_regrowth_of_hemp.pdf.

Bibliography

Org, Thecannabisindustry, and Policycouncil. 2020. "Learn More about NCIA's Policy Council ENVIRONMENTAL SUSTAINABILITY in the CANNABIS INDUSTRY IMPACTS, BEST MANAGEMENT PRACTICES, and POLICY CONSIDERATIONS." https://thecannabisindustry.org/wp-content/uploads/2020/11/NCIA-Environmental-Policy-BMP-October-17-final.pdf.

Detrano, Joseph. 2023. "Cannabis Black Market Thrives despite Legalization | Center of Alcohol & Substance Use Studies." Alcoholstudies.rutgers.edu. 2023. https://alcohol studies.rutgers.edu/cannabis-black-market-thrives-despite-legalization/.

Commentary, Guest. 2023. "Excessive Taxes, Local Control Allows California Illicit Cannabis Market to Thrive." CalMatters, June 22, 2023, sec. Commentary. https://calmatters.org/commentary/2023/06/california-illicit-cannabis-market-thrive/.

Ciara. 2023. "What Terpenes Does Gelato Have?" Caliterpenes Blog. September 29, 2023. https://www.caliterpenes.com/blog/en/what-terpenes-does-gelato-have/.

Team, RevClinics. 2022. "How THC Potency Has Changed over Time." Revolutionary Clinics. April 29, 2022. https://www.revolutionaryclinics.org/thc-potency-over-time/.

"Why Thailand Plans to Ban Recreational Weed – DW – 03/12/2024." n.d. Dw.com. Accessed April 27, 2024. https://www.dw.com/en/why-thailand-plans-to-ban-recreational-weed/video-68501590#:~:text=Since%20Thailand%20legalized%20-cannabis%20in.

Backman, I. (n.d.). Not Your Grandmother's Marijuana: Rising THC Concentrations in Cannabis Can Pose Devastating Health Risks. Medicine.yale.edu. https://medicine.yale.edu/news-article/not-your-grandmothers-marijuana-rising-thc-concentrations-in-cannabis-can-pose-devastating-health-risks/#:~:text=As%20THC%20potency%20increases%2C%20science%20fails%20to%20keep%20up&text=Over%20the%20last%20several%20decades

"Shop Delta 9 THC Products." n.d. CbdMD. Accessed July 27, 2023. https://www.cbdmd.com/collections/delta-9-thc.

Grawert, Ames. 2020. "What Is the First Step Act — and What's Happening with It? | Brennan Center for Justice." Www.brennancenter.org. June 23, 2020. https://www.brennancenter.org/our-work/research-reports/what-first-step-act-and-whats-happening-it.

National Institute of Health. (2020, February 24). RePORT. Report.nih.gov. https://report.nih.gov/funding/categorical-spending#/

Stone, E. (2022, May 18). U.S. Patent on Cannabis to Earn Millions for Government and Big Pharma. Cannabis & Tech Today. https://cannatechtoday.com/patent-on-cannabis-makes-billions-for-pharma/#:~:text=Fun%20-fact%3A%20the%20US%20Government

"The U.S. Has a Chance to Regulate Delta-8 THC. Will It?" 2023. NBC News. September 5, 2023. https://www.nbcnews.com/health/health-news/delta-8-thc-regulation-loophole-may-make-hard-know-cannabis-products-rcna102961#.

"What Is Hemp-Derived Delta-9?" n.d. Leafwell. Accessed October 21, 2023. https://leafwell.com/blog/hemp-derived-delta-9/.

Johnson, Lee. 2022. "New Study Finds over 50% of Hemp Delta-9 Products Are Mislabeled, and Stronger than Cannabis Edibles." CBD Oracle. April 26, 2022. https://cbdoracle.com/news/hemp-delta-9-thc-products-lab-study-consumer-safety-and-legality/.

"Dystonia." n.d. National Institute of Neurological Disorders and Stroke. https://www.ninds.nih.gov/health-information/disorders/dystonia#:~:text=What%20is%20dystonia%3F.

"Marijuana on the Jobsite: A Positive Test vs. Impairment." 2022. Www.nahb.org. March 16, 2022. https://www.nahb.org/blog/2022/03/marijuana-on-the-jobsite-a-positive-test-vs-impairment/.

News, M. G. H., and Public Affairs. 2022. "Harvard-Led Research Identifies Potential Test for Cannabis Impairment." Harvard Gazette. January 11, 2022. https://news.harvard.edu/gazette/story/2022/01/research-describes-brain-based-method-for-identifying-cannabis-impairment/.

Bartlett, Lindsey. n.d. "Dwyane Wade Celebrates NBA Hall of Fame Induction with Cannabis Drop." Forbes. Accessed December 8, 2023. https://www.forbes.com/sites/lindseybartlett/2023/08/14/dwyane-wade-celebrates-nba-hall-of-fame-induction-with-cannabis-drop/?sh=68af75ac47e7.

Woman, Tokin. 2019. "Tokin Woman: Top 10 Marijuana Jazz Tunes by Women." Tokin Woman. November 12, 2019. https://tokinwoman.blogspot.com/2019/11/top-10-jazz-songs-by-or-performed-by.html.

Su, Peter. 2023. "The Cannabis Industry's Efficiency Challenge: How Technology Is Leading the Way." Rolling Stone. April 11, 2023. https://www.rollingstone.com/culture-council/articles/cannabis-industrys-efficiency-challenge-how-technology-is-leading-the-way-1234712499/.

"Chris Webber on How the War on Drugs Led Him to Create a New $50M Cannabis Facility in Detroit." 2021. CBSSports.com. September 28, 2021. https://www.cbssports.com/nba/news/chris-webber-on-how-the-war-on-drugs-led-him-to-create-a-new-50m-cannabis-facility-in-detroit/.

"Marijuana and Music: Examining the Relationship." n.d. Marijuana and Music: Examining the Relationship. Accessed August 5, 2023. https://livwell.com/blog/cannabis-and-music#:~:text=Cannabis%20and%20music%20history.

Oleck, Joan. n.d. "A New 'Indigenous Cannabis Association' Aims to Unite America's Tribes around a Medicinal Plant That's Always Been with Them." Forbes. Accessed April 20, 2023. https://www.forbes.com/sites/joanoleck/2022/10/19/a-new-indigenous-cannabis-association-aims-to-unite-americas-tribes-around-a-medicinal-plant-thats-always-been-with-them/?sh=2afb7abb71a0.

Stohr, Mary K., Dale W. Willits, David A. Makin, Craig Hemmens, Nicholas P. Lovrich, Duane L. Stanton Sr., and Mikala Meize. "Effects of Marijuana Legalization on Law Enforcement and Crime: Executive Summary." Washington State University (2020). https://www.ojp.gov/pdffiles1/nij/grants/255061.pdf

Marijuana Policy Project. "Map of State Marijuana Laws," last modified May 2021. https://www.mpp.org/issues/legalization/map-of-state-marijuana-laws/

Bailey, Maggie. "Criminal Justice System Impacts of Cannabis Decriminalization & Legalization," UNC School of Government (2021). https://cjil.sog.unc.edu/wp-content/uploads/sites/19452/2021/06/Impacts-of-Cannabis-Decriminalization-Legalization-6.24.2021.pdf

Hartman, Michael. "Cannabis Overview." National Conference of State Legislatures. April 8, 2021. https://www.ncsl.org/research/civil-and-criminal-justice/marijuana-overview.aspx

Farley, Erin Jennifer, and Stan Orchowsky. "Measuring the Criminal Justice System Impacts of Marijuana Legalization and Decriminalization Using State Data." JRSA, Justice Research and Statistics Association, (2019). https://www.ojp.gov/pdffiles1/nij/grants/253137.pdf

Charles William Hobley (1902). Eastern Uganda: An Ethnological Survey. Anthropological Institute of Great Britain and Ireland. pp. 30

"Zimbabwe legalises marijuana for medical and scientific use". The Telegraph. 28 April 2018.

"Malawi ready to produce cannabis for industrial and medicinal use". Reuters. 2020-11-24.

Archive, View Author, Follow on Twitter, and Get author RSS feed. 2023. "ER Visits Spiked for Children Sickened by Cannabis during Pandemic: CDC." July 14, 2023. https://nypost.com/2023/07/13/er-visits-spiked-for-children-sickened-by-cannabis-during-pandemic-cdc/.

"Marihuana Growers Information." 2020. Usdoj.gov. 2020. https://www.deadiversion.usdoj.gov/drugreg/marihuana.htm.

"As Amsterdam Bows Out, What Will Be the New Capital of Cannabis Tourism?" 2023. Travel. September 7, 2023. https://www.nationalgeographic.com/travel/article/amsterdam-marijuana-ban-cannabis-tourism.

Wikipedia Contributors. 2019. "Drug Policy of the Netherlands." Wikipedia. Wikimedia Foundation. January 24, 2019. https://en.wikipedia.org/wiki/Drug_policy_of_the_Netherlands.

"U.S. Cannabis Market Size, Share & Growth Report, 2030." n.d. Www.grandviewresearch.com. Accessed April 27, 2024. https://www.grandviewresearch.com/industry-analysis/us-cannabis-market#:~:text=The%20US%20cannabis%20market%20size.

Johnson, Arianna. n.d. "NBA Will No Longer Penalize Marijuana Use, Report Says: Here's How Other Leagues Measure Up." Forbes. Accessed March 27, 2023. https://www.forbes.com/sites/ariannajohnson/2023/04/03/nba-will-no-longer-penalize-marijuana-use-report-says-heres-how-other-leagues-measure-up/?sh=7c5832c556d4.

"What Is Sinsemilla | Sinsemilla Definition by Weedmaps." n.d. Weedmaps. https://weedmaps.com/learn/dictionary/sinsemilla.

Bennett, Patrick. 2018. "What Are Cannabis Flavonoids and What Do They Do?" Leafly. February 9, 2018. https://www.leafly.com/news/cannabis-101/what-are-marijuana-flavonoids.

Maynes, Charles, Bill Chappell, and Rachel Treisman. 2022. "A Russian Court Sentences WNBA Star Brittney Griner to 9 Years on Drug Charges." NPR, August

4, 2022, sec. Europe. https://www.npr.org/2022/08/04/1115541890/brittney-griner-russia-drug-trial.

Maynes, Charles, Bill Chappell, and Rachel Treisman. 2022. "A Russian Court Sentences WNBA Star Brittney Griner to 9 Years on Drug Charges." NPR, August 4, 2022, sec. Europe. https://www.npr.org/2022/08/04/1115541890/brittney-griner-russia-drug-trial.

Cervantes, Jorge (2006). Marijuana horticulture: the indoor/outdoor medical grower's bible (Rev. ed.). Van Patten Pub. pp. 81. ISBN 978-1-878823-23-6. OCLC 64708236.

García, Jacobo. 2022. "Caro Quintero, El Viejo Capo Que Revolucionó El Mundo de La Marihuana." El País México. July 17, 2022. https://elpais.com/mexico/2022-07-17/caro-quintero-el-viejo-capo-que-revoluciono-el-mundo-de-la-marihuana.html.

Learning, Advanced. n.d. "Cannabis Concentrates vs Extracts vs Separations." Accessed April 27, 2024. https://www.theoriginalresinator.com/blog/cannabis-concentrates-vs-extracts/#:~:text=The%20main%20difference%20between%20a.

Desjardins, J. (2019, March 9). The 6,000-Year History of Medical Cannabis. Visual Capitalist. https://www.visualcapitalist.com/history-medical-cannabis-shown-one-giant-map/

Cartwright, M. 2017. "Paper in Ancient China." World History Encyclopedia. Mark Cartwright. September 15, 2017. https://www.worldhistory.org/article/1120/paper-in-ancient-china/.

Lawler, A. 2019. "Oldest Evidence of Marijuana Use Discovered in 2500-Year-Old Cemetery in Peaks of Western China." Science. https://www.science.org/content/article/oldest-evidence-marijuana-use-discovered-2500-year-old-cemetery-peaks-western-china#:~:text=In%20440%20B.C.E.%2C%20the%20Greek,muse-um%20in%20Stavropol%2C%20Russia%2C%20in

De Materia Medica: Being an Herbal with many other medicinal materials, translated by Tess Anne Osbaldeston (2000). (Publisher Ibidis Press: Johannesburg).

Rice, Chris. "Cannabis: A Lost History (Full Documentary)." YouTube, January 4, 2018. https://www.youtube.com/watch?v=X2p6qFT_Zjg.

"California Cannabis Tax Revenues Steered to Police Dept. Budgets." n.d. Public Health Institute. https://www.phi.org/thought-leadership/california-cannabis-tax-revenues-a-windfall-for-law-enforcement-or-an-opportunity-for-healing-communities/#:~:text=The%20revenue%20collected%20from%20cannabis.

Murray, Jon. 2018. "Cautious Approach on Marijuana Legalization Has Reaped Millions to Help Aurora's Homeless." The Denver Post. The Denver Post. December 28, 2018. https://www.denverpost.com/2018/12/28/aurora-marijuana-taxes-benefits-homeless/.

Barcott, Bruce, and Beau Whitney. 2021. "The US Cannabis Industry Now Supports 321,000 Full-Time Jobs." Leafly. February 16, 2021. https://www.leafly.com/news/industry/cannabis-jobs-report.

Herrington, A. J. n.d. "New Cannabis Jobs Report Reveals Marijuana Industry's Explosive Employment Growth." Forbes. Accessed January 21, 2024. https://www.forbes.

com/sites/ajherrington/2022/02/23/new-cannabis-jobs-report-reveals-marijuana-industrys-explosive-employment-growth/?sh=5c6e15623f2a.

"End the War on Drugs." n.d. American Civil Liberties Union. https://www.aclu.org/issues/smart-justice/sentencing-reform/end-war-drugs.

Veterans Walk And Talk. n.d. "Veterans Walk and Talk." Veterans Walk and Talk. Accessed April 27, 2023. https://veteranswalkandtalk.com.

"Veterans Action Council." n.d. VAC. Accessed July 11, 2023. https://www.veteransactioncouncil.com.

"President Biden Signs Bill Clearing the Way for Medical Cannabis Research | Advisories." n.d. Arnold & Porter. https://www.arnoldporter.com/en/perspectives/advisories/2022/12/medical-cannabis-research.

"Terry v. United States." n.d. Constitutional Accountability Center. Accessed June 22, 2023. https://www.theusconstitution.org/litigation/terry-v-united-states/#:~:text=The%20US%20Court%20of%20Appeals.

McDermott, Alicia. 2016. "Researchers Unlock the Mystery of the Mummified Lung of a Merovingian Queen." Ancient Origins Reconstructing the Story of Humanity's Past. April 20, 2016. https://www.ancient-origins.net/news-history-archaeology/researchers-unlock-mystery-mummified-lung-merovingian-queen-005744.

"Legal and Illegal Cannabis: A Cause for Growing Environmental Concern." 2022. Mongabay Environmental News. June 2, 2022. https://news.mongabay.com/2022/06/legal-and-illegal-cannabis-a-cause-for-growing-environmental-concern/.

"Sustainability in the Cannabis Industry." n.d. Https://Askgrowers.com/. https://askgrowers.com/special-project/sustainability-in-the-cannabis-industry.

Byrne, Genevieve. 2023. "Energy and Equity in Cannabis Cultivation." https://farmandenergyinitiative.org/wp-content/uploads/2023/03/FEI-CannabisReport-Final.pdf.

"SUPREME COURT of the UNITED STATES." 2020. https://www.supremecourt.gov/opinions/20pdf/20-5904_i4dk.pdf.

"Universidad Nacional Autónoma de México (UNAM)-Publicación." n.d. Hndm.iib.unam.mx. Accessed October 14, 2023. https://hndm.iib.unam.mx/consulta/publacion/visualizar/558a37d87d1ed64f16df1668?intPagina=1&tipo=pagina&palabras=marihuana&anio=1901&mes=02&dia=16.

"The Indian Hemp," The Western Journal of Medicine and Surgery, May 1843

Gordon, Cyrus: Before Columbus: Links Between the Old World & Ancient America; 1971, Crown Books, NY

Mertz, Henriette: Pale Ink: Two Ancient Records of Chinese Exploration of America; 1953/1972, Swallow Press, Chicago.

Washington, George: The Diaries of George Washington; 1925, Houghton Mifflin.

Holmes, W. H.: 13th Annual Report, Smithsonian Inst., Bur. of Ethnology (1891-1892); "Prehistoric Textile Art of the Eastern United States".

Object, object. n.d. "Cannabis Cures: American Medicine, Mexican Marijuana, and the Origins of the War on Weed, 1840-1937." Core.ac.uk. Accessed May 03, 2023. https://core.ac.uk/reader/151481330.

Humanities, National Endowment for the. 1917. "Arizona Republican. [Volume] (Phoenix, AZ) 1890-1930, May 17, 1917, Image 7." Chroniclingamerica.loc.gov,

Bibliography

May 17, 1917. https://chroniclingamerica.loc.gov/lccn/sn84020558/1917-05-17/ed-1/seq-7/.

"Is the Word 'Marijuana' Racist." n.d. The Drug Page. Accessed April 27, 2024. https://www.thedrugpage.org/racism-marijuana-nomenclature.

Rivas, Rebecca, Missouri Independent May 2, and 2023. 2023. "Why Some People Believe 'Marijuana' Is a Racist Word, and Why It Doesn't Offend Me • Missouri Independent." Missouri Independent. May 2, 2023. https://missouriindependent.com/2023/05/02/why-some-people-believe-marijuana-is-a-racist-word-and-why-it-doesnt-offend-me/.

"Robert Nelson: A History of Hemp (Chapter 2)." n.d. Www.rexresearch.com. Accessed February 19, 2023. http://www.rexresearch.com/hhist/hhist2.htm#natives.

Wikipedia Contributors. 2019. "Bering Strait." Wikipedia. Wikimedia Foundation. March 13, 2019. https://en.wikipedia.org/wiki/Bering_Strait.

"A History of Weed: From Jefferson to Clinton to Washington." 2012. MPR News. December 6, 2012. https://www.mprnews.org/story/2012/12/06/history-of-weed#.

Gieringer, Dale H. 1999. "The Forgotten Origins of Cannabis Prohibition in California." Contemporary Drug Problems 26 (2): 237–88. https://doi.org/10.1177/009145099902600204.

MANDEL NGAN/AFP via Getty Images. 2022. "Don't Expect Mass Prison Releases from Biden's Marijuana Clemency." The Marshall Project. October 15, 2022. https://www.themarshallproject.org/2022/10/15/don-t-expect-mass-prison-releases-from-biden-s-marijuana-clemency.

Schmidt, Nadine. 2024. "Germany Legalizes Recreational Cannabis Use." CNN. February 23, 2024. https://www.cnn.com/2024/02/23/europe/germany-cannabis-legal-parliament-intl/index.html.

"Zambia legalizes cannabis, kind of". The GrowthOp. 2019-12-16. https://www.thegrowthop.com/cannabis-news/zambia-legalizes-cannabis-kind-of

"Germany Legalises Cannabis: Could It Become a 'Weed Tourism' Hotspot?" 2024. Euronews. April 2, 2024. https://www.euronews.com/travel/2024/04/02/germany-legalises-cannabis-where-does-the-rest-of-europe-stand-on-weed-tourism.

Cca. 2022. "Weed Measurements: Everything You Need to Know." Cca. July 11, 2022. https://cca2go.com/weed-measurements-how-much-is-an-eighth-quarter-ounce-and-more/#:~:text=Additionally%2C%20it%20is%20considered%20the.

Acknowledgments

This work would not have been possible without the support of my community, and industry colleagues. I am especially indebted to Terri Best; Jeanmar Levi, Zoe Wilder; Savina Monet; and my sisters, Johanny, and Rafaela, who have been supportive of my career goals and who work actively to provide me with the encouragement I needed to pursue anything I set my mind to.

I am grateful to all of those with whom I have had the pleasure to work with during this and other related projects. I would especially like to thank E. Duane Alexander, my business partner and mentor, who has taught me more than I could ever give him credit for here. He has shown me, by his example, how to navigate the cannabis industry with tenacity and integrity.

I would like to thank my mother, whose love and guidance are with me in whatever I pursue. She is the ultimate role model. Most importantly, I wish to thank God for everything.

...Major props to the cannabis plant!

About the Author

JM Balbuena is legal cannabis compliance subject matter expert and business consultant. She is the founder of Synergy, a full-service cannabis industry consulting firm, and is the creator of Boycott Shitty Weed™, a cannabis advocacy lifestyle brand. She currently serves as CMO at Prime Harvest, a tech-retail focused cannabis organization and parent company to San Diego's cannabis retail dispensary and delivery platform, Jaxx Cannabis. Balbuena is the author of the Amazon bestselling book, The Successful Canna-Preneur, which is also available in Spanish. JM is a US Navy veteran and proud Afro-Latina who lives in San Diego, California.

About Synergy Studios

Synergy, is a creative endeavor born from a passion for storytelling and a commitment to the burgeoning cannabis industry. As a multimedia production company, we craft compelling content that speaks to the heart of cannabis culture. More than a business, Synergy is a movement to inspire and empower.

Other Books by JM Balbuena

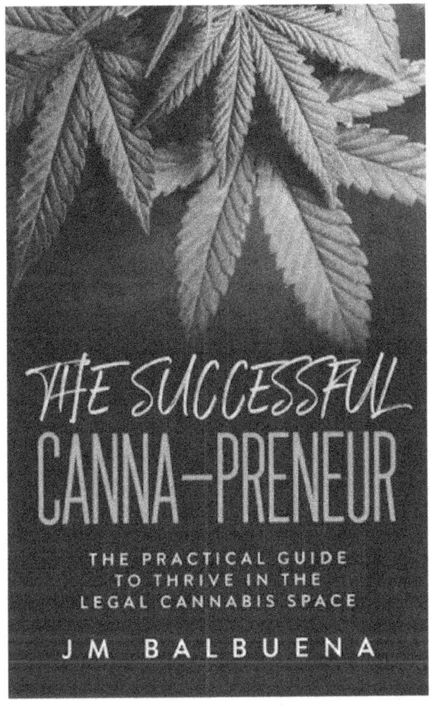

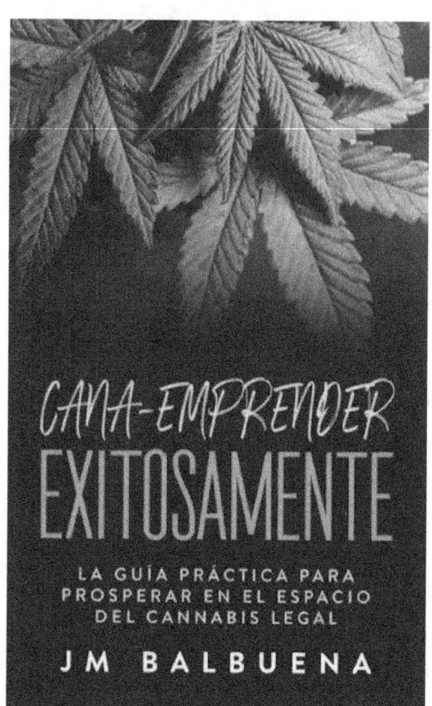

CANA-EMPRENDER
EXITOSAMENTE
LA GUÍA PRÁCTICA PARA
PROSPERAR EN EL ESPACIO
DEL CANNABIS LEGAL
JM BALBUENA

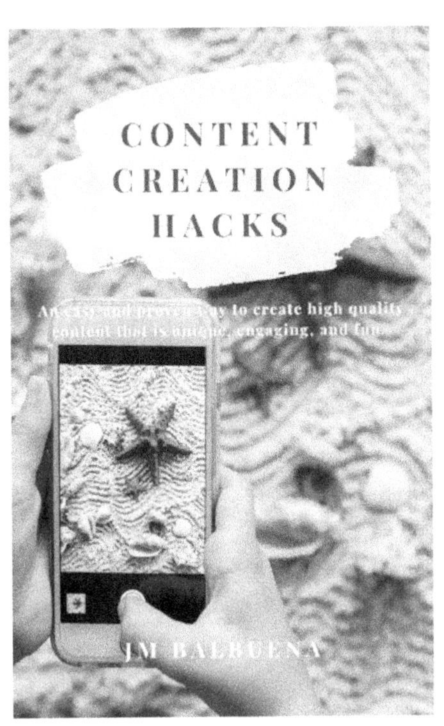

CONTENT
CREATION
HACKS
An easy and proven way to create high quality content that is unique, engaging, and fun.
JM BALBUENA

Thank You.
www.JMBalbuena.com